The Weekend Warrior

Balancing Sport, Family & Full Time Work

Mr. Will Moore

Copyright

Copyright © 2024 by Will Moore
All rights reserved.

No part of this publication may be copied, stored in a retrieval system, or transmitted in any form or by any means – electronic, mechanical, photocopying, recording, or otherwise – without the prior written permission of the author, except for brief quotations used in reviews or permitted under copyright law.

The cover photo and all contents of this book are the intellectual property of **Will Moore**. The cover photo is used exclusively with his permission and is protected under copyright law.

Moore Performance Ltd.
30 Edison Road, St Ives
Cambridge
PE27 3LF

Testimonials

If I had a very expensive classic car with a problem, I would want and search out the very best man for the job who would know to the very smallest detail how every part performed. Well, I don't have the car, but I did have a leg with a problem which to me is just as precious. So, I searched and found Will, who knows to the very smallest detail how every part performs.

A truly nice guy, put me at ease, explained the issue in a way I understood and fixed my problem.

Keith Salmon

I wish I had found Moore Performance (and in particular, Will) sooner because then I wouldn't have ended up in the pain I did. I had been seeing a local osteopath and was getting nowhere with my ankle pain so I was contemplating private surgery when I came across Moore Performance. I decided to give them a go and Will has changed my life. When I first started seeing him, I had just come back from the trip of a lifetime to Death Valley and Yosemite but had been unable to fully enjoy it as I was in too much pain to walk, even with maximum dose painkillers daily. Having previously run two marathons, it was highly upsetting to have reached the point where I couldn't even walk down my stairs or to the local shops. Will reassured me that there wasn't anything wrong with me that wasn't fixable (the GP had told me a quite different story!) and he got to work. Just under a year later and I was able to walk up the aisle to get married and also enjoy walking thousands of steps round Disney World without any pain. I have also started hiking up hills again and also playing tennis. I cannot thank Will enough for changing my life and giving me back the things I enjoy in life!

Mandy Quinney

I had a nasty knee injury. Thankfully I contacted Moore Performance in St Ives and from the first appointment 7 days after my Injury to the time I was match fit and ready to continue my international veterans football career guided me all the way back to full fitness.

The care advice professionalism and friendly service was first class though I of course had to do hours of rehabilitation and training to get back to full fitness this would not have been possible without Moore performance.

I have just played 3 games in a week for Team GB at an over 50 veterans tournament this would not have happened without you guys so thank you.

Andy Cranch

I have had issues with my calves on and off for a number of years and got to a stage that rest alone was not enough went to see Will and he identified my problem virtually straight away and after only three sessions with him I started running again am following his advice and all is still good was well worth the visit and would have no problem recommending him to anyone.

Ben Petriello

I'm really pleased that someone suggested Moore Performance to me & really pleased that they had someone who could help with my plantar fasciitis. Although I'd had plantar before it had never really been too much of a problem but this time it was so bad that I could not put my foot to the floor when I woke up in the mornings & it was so painful throughout the day too. I love walking & it stopped me from doing this as it was just so painful. I'm happy to say that after 6 visits to I have now been able to go back to my walking & this week so far has been absolutely amazing as it seems to be back to normal.

Pauline Brunning

The folks at Moore Performance are absolutely excellent. Originally, I came in for help with muscle imbalances and some niggles (shin splints at the time) when I was starting to ramp up my running, having not even ran a half marathon at this point. The in depth muscle assessments to iron our weaknesses, and the plans and programmes for strength and mobility work have been invaluable from the team. On top of this they've fixed things like joint mobilisation when I've put a lot of stress on my legs.

Fast forward a year, with their support and guidance, I have just finished my first Marathon with my legs intact, with an Ultramarathon coming up soon. Running up to this huge training block I ramped up my massage sessions with Moore Performance and bought the gold package, which I'd recommend to anyone who needs regular treatment. It's given me peace of mind they can be my go-to whenever I need anything at short notice.

If you're thinking about ironing out niggles or weaknesses, have a current injury, or just need a massage - stop holding off and book in.

Matt Jackson

The best around, high quality & professional service. Will has helped me with various different injuries and has got me back out on the pitch each time!

Chris Newton

I found that Will while treating an MCL injury was both knowledgeable and empathetic. This I am sure was in no small measure due to his time spent as a physio in a professional sports environment with both Gloucester RFC and the London Broncos. I would have no hesitation in recommending him.

Rod Dominy

I have nothing but praise for Moore Performance Ltd. All the staff are very professional and friendly, they always make you welcome and help whenever they can. I have acupuncture regularly and this treatment has kept my joints working and means that I do not have to resort to any form of medication which is important to me. I have no hesitation whatsoever in recommending them.

Audrey Drummey

I cannot recommend Will Moore (and his wider team!) highly enough! His expertise and dedication to his craft are truly exceptional. From the moment I walked into his clinic, I felt at ease. Will's thorough understanding of the human body, combined with his personalised approach, meant that my treatment was not only effective but also tailored specifically to my needs.

He took the time to listen to my concerns, explain the underlying issues, and outline a clear plan for recovery. Thanks to his guidance and support, I've made remarkable progress. What sets Will apart is his genuine care for his patients; he goes above and beyond to ensure that each session is productive and that I leave feeling better than when I arrived.

If you're looking for a someone who is professional, knowledgeable, and truly invested in your wellbeing, Will Moore is the one to see. I'm grateful to have found such a skilled practitioner and couldn't be happier with the results. If Carlsberg did therapists, then Will would be the perfect model!

Paul Humphreys

I have been treated by Will for spasm in my back. This was the result of an old injury. Previous treatments by physios and osteopaths have relieved my symptoms. The difference with Will was that he helped me understand the root of the problem. When he treated me he left a tiny amount of tension where the problem originated. Now I notice that tension arising, and am able to manage it so the back doesn't go into spasm. A life changing difference in approach!

David Lee

My son has been treated by Will over the course of a number of years now, through all his sporting injuries. Will is not only extremely knowledgeable, but my son trusts him and listens to him. He gives him realistic exercises and targets and advises on his training and match schedules when in recovery. In between appointments he is always on the end of an email to give advice and support as well. Brilliant service thank you.

Nicky Smerdon-Goodman

Dedication

This is a huge achievement that has taken 3-4 years. To get this book from an idea in my head to being published and making its way to you took a whole community; there are a lot of people who have helped me get here.

Thank you to my amazing family who are always by my side and who support me in everything I do! Thank you to Mum and Dad; you have brought me up to become who I am today, with the values and ambitions to follow this path that I am on. Thank you, Dad, you have given me so much support and knowledge in building the business and you continue to be a sounding board, always. A huge thank you to my partner, Libby, who is always there to listen to all my ambitions and ideas – which normally end with me saying "this time next year we'll be..." *(Only fools and horses quote)*. You are always by my side to make me smile and you remind me of "why" I am building this business: to give us a fantastic life full of opportunities, fun, and laughter.

Thank you to my team at Moore Performance for supporting my vision to help as many people as possible. I would not be able to help this many people on my own and would not have had the time to write this book without a great team to ensure the clinics continue to grow.

Thank you, Paul Gough, my business coach/mentor. The Mastermind community that you have created has not only provided me with the tactics and skills to build up a healthcare business, but more importantly, they've helped me develop personally to reach the goals I have. The community of coaches and members has been invaluable in building up my business, being a support network for all the challenges and successes.

Thank you, Chris, for keeping me accountable and making sure it didn't stay on my to-do-list any longer!

Thank you, Ashley, for editing this book. If anyone has read a draft email from me, or anything that has gone out without proofreading, you will know it would have been a big challenge to just understand my horrendous spelling and grammar.

Thank you, Lewis, for creating the book cover; I think it is fantastic!

Thank you to Paul Cox for taking the photo of me for the cover.

This book is for you all.

Thank you!

Table of Contents

COPYRIGHT	2
TESTIMONIALS	4
DEDICATION	9
TABLE OF CONTENTS	11
ABOUT THE AUTHOR	14
INTRODUCTION	20
What is a "Weekend Warrior"?	21
CHAPTER 1: THE BIGGEST MISTAKE WEEKEND WARRIORS MAKE	23
Mindset	23
Take Your Job Into Account	25
Not Using Time Effectively	27
Overtraining	29
Prevention is Better Than Cure	31
Ignoring Issues, Avoiding Treatment, and Taking Pain Killers	32
Things Change - Research	36
CHAPTER 2: MINDSET – HOW TO WIN THE MIND GAME	40
The Fight or Flight Response	40
The Pygmalion Effect	43
It is not the Situation; It Is How You Handle It	46
How we Think, Feel, and React	47
"We Didn't Fail... We Have Just Learnt Something That Doesn't Work."	47
How to Handle Pressure	48
Instant Versus Delayed Gratification	51
Habits	55
CHAPTER 3: TIME MANAGEMENT	58
Know Where You Are	59
Does Your Time Reflect Your Priorities?	60
Quantity And Quality Are Different Things	61
Multitasking is Overrated	62
Being Accountable	63
Make Use of Travel Time	64
Pass on Low Outcome Tasks	65
Plan Time to Recharge/Recover	67
Learn to Say No	67

KNOW WHEN TO FINISH... 68

CHAPTER 4: INJURY PREVENTION 70

IT IS IMPOSSIBLE TO PREVENT ALL INJURIES.. 70
THE REQUIREMENT OF THE SPORT 71
WHAT IF I DO MORE THAN ONE SPORT? 73
SCREENING 74
PROGRAM BUILDING 77
TECHNIQUE 78
COMPLIANCE... 79
RE-TEST 79
CROSS TRAINING 81
CROSS TRAINING FOR KIDS 83
HOW TO CROSS TRAIN 84
3D PRINTED ORTHOTICS 84
ORTHOPAEDIC PILLOWS AND MATTRESSES.. 87

CHAPTER 5: INJURY TREATMENT 94

MYTHS AND MISTAKES... 94
DEFINITION OF AN INJURY 94
UNDERSTAND THE PROBLEM YOURSELF... 95
DIAGNOSING AN INJURY 96
WHO TO SEE 96
NHS/ PRIVATE 99
SCANS... 101
X-RAY 102
ULTRASOUND 102
MAGNETIC RESONANCE IMAGING (MRI).. 102
COMPUTED TOMOGRAPHY (CT) 103
TREATMENT PLAN 107
SURGERY, INJECTIONS: THE LAST RESORT 108
GETTING IN FRONT OF THE CORRECT PERSON 109

CHAPTER 6: REHABILITATION 112

THE STAGES OF REHABILITATION 112
THE EARLY STAGE 113
POLICE 114
THE INTERMEDIATE STAGE 115
THE LATE STAGE 116
THE RETURN TO TRAINING STAGE 117
THE PREVENTION STAGE.. 118
PRINCIPLES OF REHABILITATION 119
REHAB DOESN'T STOP WHEN YOU ARE FIT TO COMPETE 121

CHAPTER 7: TRAINING METHODS 124

SPORTS/EVENT SPECIFIC TRAINING... 124

- Speed Training 126
- Cardiovascular Endurance 128
- Change of Direction and Agility 130
- Gym/Strength Training 131
- Coordination/Reaction 133
- Flexibility/Mobility 134
- Cross-Training 136
- Tactical/Analysis 137
- Mental/Psychological Training 139

CHAPTER 8: RECOVERY STRATEGIES 142

- Do the Simple Things Well 143
- Planning 144
- Engaging 144
- Stretching and Mobility 145
- Hydrotherapy 147
- Sleep 149
- The Pillow Matters 153
- Nutrition 155
- Hydration 156
- Ice baths/Cryotherapy 158
- Cryotherapy Chambers 161
- Compression 162

CHAPTER 9: CONCLUSION – BRINGING IT ALL TOGETHER 166

- Your Journey as a Weekend Warrior 171

WHAT'S NEXT 173

REFERENCES 176

About the Author

Who Is Cambridgeshire's Leading Sports Injuries Expert, Will Moore?

I was born and raised in St. Ives Cambridgeshire (not to be confused with the St Ives in Cornwall). My family has lived in this town for decades and still do. In fact, my grandparents used to own a sweet shop in the town, so we've always had businesses here and continue to enjoy a presence in the local community.

I had always been sports-mad growing up, I would try any sport that I came across my path. My main passion is rugby. When I'm not working in the field, I love to watch it. Of course, I used to play rugby when I was a kid – from the age of 10 until after university – but the demands of a professional career in the sport led me to focus solely on my job. During my free time, though, you'll often see me at my local rugby club St. Ives RFC. It's where I played as a kid, and I still have great memories of that club. I'll always support them. Up The Ives!!

I have grown up around business: my grandparents had a newsagents/sweet shop, as I mentioned. Some of my earliest memories involve helping my grandad serve the newspapers behind the counter and helping stock up the sweets and ice creams. It was probably inevitable that, one day, I would have a business of my own.

With great help from my Dad (Adrian) and business coach Paul Gough, I have grown from working part-time for myself to having a multi-clinic business with a number of staff. I am always looking for what is next. My greatest desire is to help more people whilst giving my family a fantastic, fun, loving, and safe life that is full of opportunities and new experiences.

In fact, I am now in a position where I am able to offer other people, especially business owners, advice on how to succeed and grow. Admittedly, it is a very unusual feeling; I am very far from the finished article and I am constantly learning and growing myself, but it is extremely rewarding when I am now able to help people in a number of different ways.

I started my career in professional rugby union and league, working with various professional rugby teams. I did that for 5 years, but then decided to move on to something different. The reality is, my job in professional sport was taking too much out of me; I was constantly travelling with sports teams. That's when the idea struck me – *why not establish a clinic where the expertise and skills I've acquired working with elite athletes could be accessible to everyone?* I wanted to extend the same level of care, knowledge, and individualised treatment plans to anyone looking for it without being encumbered by vast amounts of travel and time lost. Therefore, I founded my first clinic in St. Ives, Cambridgeshire, and to this day we offer services similar to those provided to professional sports teams.

Many people might remember seeing me during my time working in professional rugby. I had the privilege of working with teams primarily in Premiership Rugby and Super League. Actually, you might have seen me rushing onto the pitch during games, especially if there was an injury on the field. There is nothing better than being part of a rugby team for a big game that is live on Sky Sports. In rugby, the medical team have a lot of work to do; there would be a number of players that would not be on that pitch if it wasn't for the medical team. The pressure and energy of a match-day is very unique and something that I absolutely loved. The feeling of standing pitch side knowing you are looking after a number of players' safety, especially as you are being watched and scrutinised by the commentators and keyboard worriers, does take a lot planning and training; it is not for everyone, but I thrived under the pressure –being part of the team's highs and lows os a real roller coaster ride.

The last professional club which I worked for, The London Broncos Rugby League Club, will always hold for me some of the best memories from both a career point of view and personally.

Thank you to Dan Watson, the Head of Medical, who brought me into the club; we had some incredible times as a medical team and we then great friends. One memory that springs to mind is the million-pound game. It was the play-off final to get to the Super League and we were playing against Toronto Wolfpack in Canada. We didn't expect to get there, but the week before we won the play-off, which meant there was an incredible rush to get everything ready to fly to Canada with a few days' notice. It was the end of a very tough season, so we already had quite a few players who were battered and bruised. Therefore, we had our work cut out to get them on the pitch.

We managed to get a few players who were very unlikely to make it out onto the pitch and play the game. We went in as extreme underdogs, but we went on to win by a couple of points. It was incredible to have played a part in that achievement for the club. I always had a great time working for the Broncos, and the rest of the coaching staff created the best club atmosphere that I have been a part of. We overcame lots of adversity, had great medical successes, as well as fantastic experiences with a few beers, snacks and stories along the way.

My business is called Moore Performance. At present, I have a network of 3 clinics with a number of great staff. We offer athletes and active people the resources to live pain-free and carry on with their lives. At Moore Performance, my mission is to help as many people as possible. Sport is my passion and my life. If I'm not fixing sports injuries, I'm watching sports.

All-in-all, because of my passion for sport and for people, I help individuals who prioritise fitness to enhance their activity levels without reliance on pain medication. Enhancement is therefore a large part of what we do at my clinics, but we also treat pain.

At Moore Performance we treat everything from simple aches and pains to very complex traumatic injuries and everything in between. We tailor our approach to each individual because we know everyone is different; your goals are different, so why wouldn't your plan of care be different? We ensure you know exactly what the issues are in straightforward, non-complex language, and we explain the steps you need to take to achieve your goals.

I started in this industry for a number of reasons. The first is that helping people is really important to me. I am very passionate about helping others, and what better way to help people than assisting them to become more active and pain-free? The second is that during my rugby career, I unfortunately had a lot of injuries; these ultimately led to being a big factor in my personal decision to stop playing rugby. Back then, there wasn't as much research or information available as you'll find in this book: if I had the knowledge that I have now, I might not have had to retire.

So, a big goal of mine is for people not to have to stop sport like I had to.

My journey also means that I have had first-hand experience with several different types of injuries and, therefore, various different treatment plans over the years – from operations to electrotherapy, through to orthotics and rehab. I've been through it personally. This personal experience has been invaluable, and some of the people I met through my injuries have inspired me to go down this route.

So, we are a sports injury business – that is our specialty. Anyone who is active, in our opinion, is a sports person - you don't have to be part of a football or rugby team to be fit. We class someone as active if they do lots of walking, running, or simply keep up with their children or grandchildren. In fact, our multidisciplinary team offers diverse specialty treatment, including a focus rugby, running, and other sports, as well as expertise in specific injuries. We're confident in our ability to match you with a specialist capable of addressing your injury and aiding your recovery.

Whether it's taking a holiday, spending time with the kids, or playing sports and activities you love, an injury can impact your whole life. Many individuals, like me, have sports deeply intertwined with their lives. Weekends usually revolve around going to games or being active with friends.

Unsurprisingly, if you love a sport and you get injured, that's a big part of your free time gone. Sports injuries aren't just about the pain they cause; they disrupt your entire routine and social life, depriving you of a vital outlet from work or family responsibilities. This void is acutely felt, affecting not only physical activity but also overall well-being.

Injuries, regardless of where they occur, have repercussions beyond the pitch or the court. Even if sustained during sports and exacerbated during moderate activity, they hinder everyday tasks such as being comfortable at work or picking up your children or grandchildren.

Having deep-rooted connections in St. Ives, it is important for me to remain connected with local groups, sports teams, and gyms. As such, we help at events by having our stand set up and ready to provide sports injury assessments of any kind. We also host what we call a 'drop-in-clinic' at local gyms, where people can come in for complimentary injury advice and to see if we're the right fit for them, all without any obligation.

And whilst our presence is felt in our community, it is also quite visible on social media – we're actively engaged with several sports clubs, including the local rugby, hockey, football, and swimming clubs. We're always on the lookout for new clubs to support, especially those within our local community.

My expertise comes from working with professional athletes and people who have attended my clinic for treatment over the 7 years I have been open. Our track record speaks for itself, as evidenced by our many five-star reviews on Google and our website. These testimonials speak to the success stories of people whose problems were resolved.

I do not know what is next for me in business or in life, but I do know that it will involve helping people in pain and those who want to be more active and happier doing the things they love. If I can help business owners on their own journey, then wonderful. In all things, I believe in doing my best – that's why I wrote this book. It is my gift to you, and it is my singular hope that what you read in the following pages gives you some clarity as to what your life could be if you were pain free. I want to give you the tools to get there, and I want you to know that I will be there every step of the way.

As Dell Boy says in perhaps one of the greatest TV shows of all time, *Only Fools and Horses*,
"He who dares, Wins!". So, are you ready to take the leap with me?

Enjoy the book!

Introduction

This book is not about giving you the exact answers; that would be impossible, as everyone has different goals and obstacles. I will, however, give you ways in which you are able to get to those answers for yourself because, after all, knowledge is power.

We hear a lot about the lifestyle of professional athletes' training routines and how hard they work. For them, it is their job; their whole lives revolve around their sport. Remember, they have the infrastructure around them to help support them. In the modern world of sports, athletes in high-level sports have an abundance of highly skilled people behind them; some of these include coaches, managers, strength and conditioning coaches, sports scientists, nutritionists, physiotherapists, and doctors, to name just a few. Even eating schedules are regulated! Why? Because it is a job.

For amateur or semi-professional athletes, things are quite different. They have a significantly harder time reaching their potential in sports. Contending with a full-time job really hampers the amount of time they can spend on the proverbial field. Most sports teams train Tuesday through Thursday for an hour or so and then play a game on Sunday. The rest of the time, well, they are on their own with only Google to help.

Sound familiar?

Throughout this book, I will pass on a number of easily implemented strategies that I have picked from my years in professional sport, mixing them in with my time as a rugby player and time in semi-pro and amateur sport. It will provide you with the knowledge and strategies to make the most efficient use of your time and help you reach your sporting potential around your full-time job.

Not an athlete?

This book is not just for those who class themselves as 'athletes'. There are lots of tips and tricks that will be able to help anyone who wants to be active at any level, whether that is carrying the shopping or picking up the kids or grandkids. There is lots of information and practical tips to help you to become more active, healthy and pain-free. Whether you classify yourself as an athlete or not, it is about using your body to do what you would like to do and not comparing yourself to others.

This book is not meant to be a one-time read; it is meant to be a reference as you move into this next, elevated phase of your life. It contains a lot of information that you will be able to implement immediately in order to make a significant difference. Equally, there is a lot of information that you will need in the future as circumstances change and different hurdles are faced. **You should always focus on the strategies which are going to move the needle the most**.

Overall, I want us to go on this journey together – as you move through the pages in this book, remember that small changes make a big difference, and, as you follow the advice I give, I'm convinced you'll start to experience growth. All the very best of luck!

What is a "Weekend Warrior"?

A "Weekend Warrior" is someone who passionately pursues sport or fitness during their free time, typically on weekends, while balancing the demands of a full-time job, family, and other life responsibilities. Unlike professional athletes, who have dedicated time and resources to train, a Weekend Warrior juggles their athletic ambitions with the realities of daily life – fitting workouts and games into the limited windows of time they have available outside of work and family duties.

Despite their busy schedules, Weekend Warriors are deeply committed to their sport and activity, often pushing themselves to perform at a high level, whether it's through recreational sports, running, cycling, or participating in weekend competitions. However, their intense drive can sometimes lead to challenges, such as overtraining, injury, or burnout, especially when they don't have access to the same recovery resources and support systems as professional athletes.

In essence, a Weekend Warrior is anyone who refuses to let a busy lifestyle stop them from being active and competing. They balance their passion for fitness and sport with their responsibilities, often sacrificing sleep, relaxation, and personal time to maintain their athletic pursuits. This book, *Weekend Warrior*, is designed to help them excel in their sport while staying healthy, injury-free, and managing the delicate balance between sport, work, and life.

Chapter 1: The Biggest Mistake Weekend Warriors Make

Let's start off by talking about some of the most common mistakes that I see people make on a regular basis. Remember, if you don't know the problems you face or may potentially face down the line, how can you fix them? In fact, how can you avoid them happening in the first place if you're not sure what could happen? You may not currently be experiencing any issues or pain, but you may in the future, and that's why we need to think about what you can change in the present.

If you are trying to juggle sports around a busy work or home life, it can be a struggle to decide on what areas you should focus on and at what time. So, if you're trying to decipher this and are looking to be the best you can be with the resources you have, then you're in luck... this is the book for you.

I will go into detail about the solutions to various issues in more depth throughout the following chapters, but in the next few pages I will first go into some of the mistakes which I have seen over many years of working with professional and amateur athletes. I'm sure some – if not most – will resonate with you. When one of them does sound like something you are doing or need help with, there will be some practical tips and information to follow. So, keep reading!

Mindset

In the world of sports, success isn't solely determined by physical ability. While athleticism and skill are undoubtedly crucial, the mindset an athlete adopts can either propel them to greatness or hinder their potential.

Athletes at every level, from beginners to professionals, often make critical mistakes rooted in a poor mindset that sabotages their performance and impedes their progress. Understanding these mistakes is the first step towards overcoming them and achieving peak performance.

One of the most common mistakes athletes make is **allowing the fear of failure to control their actions and decisions**. Fear can paralyse athletes, causing them to play it safe, avoid risks, and ultimately limit their potential. Instead of embracing challenges and viewing failure as an opportunity for growth, they become fixated on avoiding mistakes at all costs. This mindset stifles creativity, innovation, and resilience, ultimately hampering progress.

Negative self-talk, characterised by self-criticism, doubt, and pessimism, can have a negative impact on an athlete's performance and confidence. When athletes constantly berate themselves or dwell on past mistakes, it undermines their self-belief and erodes their motivation. Negative self-talk can create a self-fulfilling prophecy, where athletes internalise their doubts and perform below their capabilities as a result.

Athletes with a fixed mindset believe that their abilities and talents are innate and unchangeable. They view setbacks as evidence of their limitations rather than opportunities for growth. This rigid mindset can lead to a fear of challenges, a reluctance to step outside of their comfort zone, and a lack of resilience in the face of adversity. As a result, athletes may plateau in their development and fail to reach their full potential.

Athletes often fall into the trap of fixating on outcomes such as winning or losing, at the expense of focusing on the present moment and the process of performance. When athletes become overly preoccupied with outcomes, they may become anxious, lose sight of their game plan, and underperform as a result.

Many athletes focus primarily on physical training while neglecting the importance of mental preparation. They fail to develop strategies for managing stress, maintaining focus, and staying resilient in the face of adversity. As a result, they may crumble under pressure, succumb to distractions, or lose confidence during competition.

If any of these above resonate with you, fear not. I offer valuable tips and tricks to overcome these mindset barriers in the Mindset Chapter, come up next.

Take Your Job Into Account

In the pursuit of athletic excellence, many athletes face the daunting challenge of balancing their passion for sport with the demands of a full-time job. Whether it's striving to reach the next level, or just staying fit, healthy, and active. **The struggle to fit training and performance around a nine-to-five job is a constant reality**.

Perhaps the most obvious struggle athletes face when juggling training and a full-time job is the scarcity of time. Balancing work commitments with rigorous training schedules leaves little room for rest and recovery, let alone other aspects of life such as family time and social activities. Athletes often find themselves waking up early or staying up late to squeeze in workouts, thereby sacrificing sleep and personal time in the process.

The mental strain of balancing training and work responsibilities can be significant, consequently leading to increased stress, anxiety, and cognitive fatigue. Athletes may find it challenging to stay focused, maintain motivation, and perform at their best amidst the pressures of both worlds.

The relentless demands of both training and work can take a toll on athletes' physical and mental wellbeing. Balancing intense workouts with the mental strain of a demanding job can lead to exhaustion, burnout, and decreased performance in both arenas. Moreover, athletes may struggle to maintain energy levels, recover adequately, and stay motivated amidst competing priorities.

You probably spend more time at work than you do training or taking part in your sport, but what you are *actually* doing during this time is often forgotten. I see a lot of athletes that do a number of different professions, all of which have their different requirements physically, mentally, or time-wise. It is crucial that this is taken into account. There are so many different professions out there, the traditional 9-5 desk jobs, the manual trades, shift workers, etc. Different types of jobs put very different stresses and strains on the body, all of which require that your training is modified accordingly. For example, if you are a person with a desk-based job, your body will be sedentary for most of the day and, therefore, will need to focus on mobility and movement before the intensity is built up. For a manual trade, you may be on your feet all day, lifting, moving, using your body to get into different spaces etc, therefore, will need to take into account that your body will be using a lot of energy as well a strength during the day which will effect the way in which you recover.

Start with the requirements of your job and work out what stresses it puts on your body; is it strenuous, sedentary, using lots of energy, affecting sleep, etc. Once you understand what you are putting your body through at work, you must use the tips later in this book to adjust your training and recovery to make sure they work hand in hand with your job.

Maintaining optimal nutrition and prioritising recovery are essential components of athletic performance, yet they can be challenging to manage alongside a demanding job. Athletes may struggle to plan and prepare nutritious meals, prioritise sleep and recovery, and adhere to consistent training schedules amidst the demands of work and daily life.

Not Using Time Effectively

In the demanding world of sports, the management of time is as crucial as physical conditioning or skill development. **Poor planning of time can be a subtle yet profound enemy, affecting how athletes train, perform, and recover.** Without adequate scheduling and time management, athletes may find themselves in a cycle of underperformance and inadequate recovery, which can lead to diminished results and increased risk of injury.

The consequences of poor time planning starts at training, the bedrock of all performance. Ideally, training should be systematic and progressive, allowing for the gradual build-up of fitness and skill. However, without proper time allocation, training can become erratic and unstructured. Athletes may try to cram intense sessions into a short period, thinking intensity can make up for lost time, or they may skip essential aspects of training due to a lack of time. This can lead to incomplete preparation for competitions, where skills are not fully developed; the body might not be adequately conditioned, thereby raising the likelihood of underperformance or injury.

Moreover, the ripple effects of poorly managed training schedules extend into everyday life. Athletes balancing education, jobs, or personal commitments may find themselves juggling too many responsibilities with insufficient time to dedicate to each. The stress from this balancing act can lead to mental fatigue, which is often overlooked as a performance inhibitor. Mental exhaustion can sap motivation, reduce focus during training and competitions, and increase the risk of decision-related errors in sport.

In truth, performance is directly influenced by how well athletes can execute their skills under pressure, which in turn is highly dependent on how well they have managed their time leading up to the event.

Poor time planning can lead to inadequate warm-up or preparation on the day of competition, which not only hampers performance but also increases the risk of acute injuries. Additionally, athletes who consistently find themselves pressed for time may not have ample opportunity to strategize or mentally prepare for the demands of competition, leading to increased anxiety and decreased performance.

What's more, recovery, an essential component of athletic performance, is perhaps most vulnerable to the pitfalls of poor time management. Recovery is not just about resting but involves active processes such as sleep, nutrition, hydration, and various forms of physical therapy, all of which require time. Athletes who fail to allocate time for proper recovery may experience the accumulation of fatigue, both physical and mental, which can degrade performance over time and heighten injury rates. Overlooking recovery can create a vicious cycle where the athlete is never performing at their peak due to residual fatigue and is always playing catch-up with their conditioning.

The importance of structured recovery protocols cannot be overstated. These include sleep, which must be ample and of good quality to facilitate physiological repairs and psychological well-being; nutrition, which requires time for planning, preparation, and consumption of meals that meet the energy demands of training and aid in the repair and growth of tissues; and hydration, essential for maintaining performance and metabolic health. Each of these elements needs to be carefully integrated into an athlete's schedule to optimise recovery and performance.

Psychological recovery, including stress management and relaxation, also requires careful time management. Activities such as meditation, yoga, or simply leisure time that allow mental decompression are vital for maintaining an athlete's mental health but often get side-lined due to poor time planning.

In addition to affecting individual athletes, poor time management can also impact team dynamics. Teams that fail to synchronise their schedules effectively may find less cohesion in their execution and a decrease in teamwork, leading to poor collective performance.

The management of time within a team context requires coordination of not just training and recovery, but also of strategy sessions, team meetings, and travel plans, all integral to the success of the team.

In sports where you have a coach it is important to have a good relationship with them so you can work together helping to prioritise tasks, set realistic goals, and create schedules that allow sufficient time for all aspects of training, competition, and recovery. This involves education about the interplay between all facets of preparation and performance, as well as monitoring and adjusting plans as necessary to prevent burnout.

Ultimately, the careful planning of time in sports transcends mere scheduling. It involves a holistic approach that considers the various elements critical to an athlete's success. By recognising the importance of time in training, performance, and recovery, athletes and coaches can create an environment where peak performance is not just an aspiration but a reachable goal. Poor planning of time can be the Achilles' heel for even the most talented athletes, while effective time management can elevate an athlete's career, ensuring longevity and success in the competitive world of sports.

Overtraining

People often think the more you train the more results you have, but this is not always the case. Normal fatigue leads to muscle growth and increased performance as the body adapts to cope with it, but when there's not enough recovery time and the training is too intense over a prolonged period it adversely leads to a decrease in performance and a significant increase in injury risk.

One of the most immediate consequences of overtraining is physical fatigue, which manifests as persistent feelings of tiredness, lethargy, and soreness. When athletes push their bodies beyond their limits without allowing sufficient time for rest and recovery, they deplete their energy reserves and compromise their ability to perform at peak levels. As a result, performance metrics such as strength, speed, and endurance may decline, and athletes may struggle to achieve their training goals or meet competition expectations.

In addition to physical fatigue, overtraining can also take a toll on athletes' mental and emotional well-being. The relentless demands of excessive training can lead to feelings of burnout, frustration, and disillusionment. Athletes may experience a loss of motivation, enthusiasm, and enjoyment for their sport, as well as heightened levels of stress, anxiety, and mood disturbances. Mental fatigue can impair cognitive function, concentration, and decision-making abilities, further undermining athletic performance and enjoyment of the sport.

Overtraining can disrupt the delicate balance of hormones involved in regulating metabolism, energy production, and stress response. Chronic elevations in stress hormones such as cortisol and adrenaline can lead to hormonal imbalances, metabolic dysfunction, and disturbances in sleep patterns. Poor sleep quality and inadequate restorative sleep further exacerbate the effects of overtraining, perpetuating a vicious cycle of fatigue, impaired recovery, and decreased performance. Furthermore, overtraining compromises the immune system, making athletes more susceptible to illness and infections, which can further derail training plans and delay progress towards performance goals.

Perhaps the most common consequence of overtraining is psychological burnout – a state of emotional and mental exhaustion characterised by apathy, disillusionment, and a loss of passion for the sport.

When athletes push themselves too hard, for too long, without adequate rest and recovery, they risk not only physical injury but also mental and emotional burnout. Over time, the relentless pursuit of performance goals can overshadow the intrinsic joy and satisfaction that initially drew athletes to their sport, leading to a sense of emptiness and disconnection.

Prevention is Better Than Cure

When we talk about staying healthy and avoiding injury, there's an old saying that really hits the nail on the head: "prevention is better than cure." This isn't just wise advice – it's a critical strategy for keeping ourselves safe in sports, at work, and even doing everyday chores around the house. Think about it: dealing with an injury can be a real hassle. It's not just the pain or the trip to the hospital; it's the aftermath paying for treatment, missing work, or sitting out during your favourite activities.

So, why not just avoid injuries in the first place? It makes sense on so many levels. For starters, injuries are expensive. Medical bills can pile up fast, and if you're off work you're losing money there, too. But, there's more to it. Some injuries can stick with you for life, thereby leading to long-term health problems that could have been avoided with a little foresight.

Take sports, for example. Whether you're a weekend warrior or a serious athlete, the right preparation is key. This means warming up properly, using the right equipment, and not pushing your limits too hard. In a lot of sports, coaches are crucial, here; they make sure everyone's playing it safe and not just playing hard.

Then there's work, especially if your job involves physical labour. Employers should provide the right tools and training to avoid injuries, but this is not always the case. Always aim for ergonomic desks, proper lifting techniques, and regular breaks.

Everyday life is full of injury risks too, but simple steps can make a big difference. Use a seat belt, keep your home free of tripping hazards, and maybe don't stand on a swivel chair to reach the top shelf... yes, it's common sense, but it's also effective. The last thing you want to do is not be able to play a match because you fell off a precariously balanced chair, right?

There's also a mental side to this. Getting hurt can be traumatic, therefore leading to anxiety. By avoiding injury, you're not just keeping your body safe, you're looking out for your mental health too.

But, of course, it's not always easy. Sometimes people don't know how to prevent injuries, or they think taking precautions is too expensive or time-consuming. That's where education comes in and that's where I too, for that matter, come in – and so does this book!

Ignoring Issues, Avoiding Treatment, and Taking Pain Killers

The longer you wait to deal with an injury, the worse it can get. It's like watching a small crack in your windshield slowly spider-web out into a major problem. Nobody wants that, right? So why do we often wait around, hoping that injuries will just magically heal themselves?

Ignoring an injury or putting off getting help can be a big mistake. What starts as a minor issue can quickly turn into a nightmare. For example, a simple sprained ankle can lead to more serious joint problems or even chronic pain if you don't treat it right and give it time to heal. The body is amazing at healing, but it's not invincible. It often needs help to get things right, whether that's proper rest, physical therapy, or medical treatment.

Think about professional athletes: when they get hurt, they're usually quick to get checked out and start their recovery plan. That's because they know something crucial: the sooner you address an injury, the quicker and smoother your recovery will likely be. They want to get back in the game as soon as possible, and dragging their feet could mean sitting out the whole season instead of just a game or two.

For us civilians, it's no different. Whether you've twisted your knee gardening or pulled your back moving furniture, the principle is the same. The longer you ignore the pain and avoid seeing a professional, the more you risk complicating your recovery. And, if we're being honest, chronic pain is debilitating, and not addressing it will eventually affect your mental health.

So, why do people wait? Well, sometimes it's about not wanting to admit that we're hurt. Or maybe it's the hassle of making doctor's appointments, dealing with medical bills, or taking time off work. But while these concerns are valid, they pale in comparison to the long-term damage and pain that can come from not treating an injury.

Economically speaking, it makes more sense to deal with injuries ASAP. Think about it: a quick visit to the doctor now might save you money down the road. You might avoid expensive surgeries or long-term treatments that become necessary when problems are left to fester. **Early intervention is not just good for your health – it's good for your wallet, too.**

And let's not forget the mental toll. Dealing with ongoing pain or mobility issues can be tough. It can suck the joy out of your favourite activities and even affect your mental health. The sooner you get on top of your injury, the sooner you can get back to feeling like yourself.

Now, how can we get better at this? First, we need to listen to our bodies. Pain is the body's way of saying something is wrong. Ignoring it doesn't make it go away; it's a signal that shouldn't be muted. Acknowledge it and take action.

Educating ourselves about common injuries and how to handle them can also make a big difference. Knowing the basics of first aid, when to apply ice or heat, and when to see a professional can prevent a lot of trouble. And in today's world – with so much information at our fingertips – there's really no excuse not to be informed.

So, let's break down a common scenario in sports: you're playing, you get hurt, and the first thing you reach for is a painkiller. It's almost a reflex. Eat a pill, dull the pain, and keep going. But here's the thing: while painkillers can be a quick fix to get you through the game, they're not a solution. Relying on them can actually do more harm than good.

Imagine this: you've got nagging knee pain from last week's game. You could rest it, or maybe see a physio, but instead you take some painkillers and jump right back into playing. Sure, you feel okay now, but what you're really doing is masking the problem. Under the influence of those painkillers, you might not realise that you're aggravating the injury. And just like that, a minor issue becomes a major one.

Pain is your body's way of saying, "Hey, something's wrong!" When you mask that signal with painkillers, you're basically ignoring your body's warning system. It's like turning off the smoke alarm because it's annoying, even though your house is on fire.

Athletes often feel pressure to perform, which can lead them to rely on painkillers. But the truth is that taking painkillers to continue playing can lead to a cycle of injury and re-injury, thereby making recovery even longer and more complicated. The longer an injury is ignored, the worse it can get... potentially leading to chronic issues that could have been avoided.

And what about the side effects? The regular use of painkillers, especially the stronger kinds, can damage your stomach, liver, and even your kidneys. And of course, some painkillers can be addictive which can lead to an entirely new set of problems.

So, what's a better approach? Firstly, give your body a chance to heal. This might mean taking a break from the sport; a short break now could mean a longer play later. And while you're taking that break, get the right treatment.

Getting educated about your body and how it works can also help you understand why medication isn't the best answer. Knowledge is power! The more you know about injury prevention and recovery, the better you can handle it when something does go wrong.

There's also a lot to be said for preventive measures. Proper warm-ups, strength training, and using the right equipment can all reduce the risk of injury in the first place. And if you do get injured, having a solid recovery plan that goes beyond painkillers can help you get back to your sport faster and stronger.

It's also worth mentioning that managing pain doesn't always mean medication. There are plenty of non-drug approaches that can help with pain, like acupuncture, meditation, and even certain breathing techniques. Exploring these can give you tools that help not just with injury, but with handling the everyday stress of sports.

Workplaces and sports clubs can help by creating an environment where it's okay to speak about injuries and not feel pressured to play/push through pain. Coaches and trainers should encourage this kind of openness and prioritise the health of their athletes!

So, next time you're thinking about reaching for the painkillers after an injury, consider what you might be masking. Speak with a professional, listen to your body, and give yourself the best chance to heal properly. Remember, taking care of an injury properly from the start isn't just about getting back in the game, it's about staying in the game for as long as you love it.

If you find yourself shrugging off an injury or thinking it will just get better on its own, remember that that's a risky gamble. The truth is that injuries need attention. The sooner, the better. It's not just about healing faster; it's about healing smarter and preventing hurt down the line.

Next time you get a knock, a twist, or a pull, don't just hope for the best. Get it checked out, follow through with treatment, and get back to doing what you love, pain-free and with peace of mind. That's how you play the long game in taking care of your health. And trust me, your future self will thank you for not waiting around.

Things Change - Research

In the dynamic and fast-paced realm of sports, the landscape of injury research is constantly evolving, driven by technological advancements, shifting paradigms in medical science, and an ever-deepening understanding of human physiology and biomechanics. This rapid progression underlines a critical aspect of sports science: what we know about preventing, treating, and rehabilitating sports injuries today may be significantly refined or even overhauled tomorrow. As researchers continue to delve into the intricacies of how injuries occur and the most effective methods for treatment, their findings often lead to substantial changes in protocols that directly impact athlete care.

The pace at which new insights and innovations emerge can be dizzying. Only a few decades ago, for example, the standard advice for dealing with a soft tissue injury was the RICE method: Rest, Ice, Compression, and Elevation. This approach was widely accepted as the best immediate treatment to reduce swelling and speed up recovery. However, recent studies have begun to question and refine this strategy, suggesting that some degree of movement and more specific cooling techniques may lead to more optimal outcomes. Such shifts in understanding are not merely academic; they have tangible effects on how injuries are managed at every level of sport, from amateur to professional teams.

Technological advancements play a huge role in driving these changes. Innovations in imaging technology, such as MRI and ultrasound, have greatly enhanced our ability to accurately diagnose the nature and extent of injuries. Wearable technology, including motion sensors and biometric monitors, now allows for real-time data collection on an athlete's biomechanics and physiological responses during both training and competition. This influx of data has not only improved our understanding of what causes injuries but also how they can be prevented through personalised training regimens and equipment adjustments.

Additionally, integrating big data analytics and machine learning into sports injury research has opened up new frontiers. These technologies can analyse vast amounts of data from diverse sources including training loads, recovery rates, and even genetic information to identify patterns that may predict injury risks. As a result, interventions can become more proactive rather than reactive, fundamentally changing the approach to injury prevention and athlete management.

The influence of evolving research is also evident in the rehabilitation processes. Advances in physical therapy, such as the development of new therapeutic exercises, electrostimulation, and regenerative medicine techniques like stem cell therapy, platelet-rich plasma (PRP) treatments, and shockwave therapy, are reshaping recovery protocols. These methods could promise quicker restoration of function and better long-term outcomes, reducing the time athletes spend side-lined and potentially extending their careers.

Furthermore, the shift towards a more holistic approach to athlete health is a significant change in sports medicine, one which is influenced by recent research. There is a growing recognition of the importance of mental health in the recovery process, leading to integrated care strategies that address psychological as well as physical aspects of recovery. Sports psychologists and mental health professionals are becoming regular members of sports medical teams, emphasising the importance of mental resilience and a positive mindset in overcoming injury.

Nutritional science has also seen substantial advancements that impact injury recovery and prevention. The understanding of how certain nutrients affect tissue repair and muscle recovery has led to more sophisticated dietary recommendations tailored to support specific recovery needs. This nutritional approach not only speeds up recovery but also enhances overall performance, showing the interconnected nature of diet, health, and athletic achievement.

The legal and ethical dimensions of sports injury research are also evolving rapidly. As more is understood about the long-term consequences of injuries – particularly brain injuries in contact sports – organisations face increasing pressure to prioritise safety over competitive success. This has led to changes in rules and equipment standards, as well as how injuries are reported and managed. The push from legal and ethical standpoints is ensuring that sport governing bodies and teams are more accountable for athlete welfare.

The rapid changes in sports injury research demands ongoing education and adaptation among healthcare professionals, trainers, and coaches. It's a field where lifelong learning isn't just beneficial but essential. **Athletes and medical professionals need to stay current with the latest research developments and be willing to adjust their practices based on the latest evidence in order to provide the best care possible and to minimise and manage injuries effectively.**

The field of sports injury research is marked by continual advancements. Each new discovery or technological breakthrough has the potential to significantly alter the understanding of sports injuries and reshape prevention and treatment strategies. For you, staying informed about these changes can mean the difference between an injury and a timely return to play. For medical professionals, it demands a commitment to continuous learning and adaptability. The only constant in the world of sports injury research is change, and embracing this dynamic nature is crucial for anyone involved in the field of sports health.

This chapter has looked at some of the most common pitfalls many amateur athletes tend to succumb to. As we move into the next chapter, I'll start to uncover techniques you can use to mitigate the effect of the above, but also to avoid them all together as you continue your training.

Let's keep going.

Throughout this book, you'll find strategies and insights to help you excel in your sport while balancing the demands of life. But that's not all: by scanning the QR code provided below and throughout, you'll gain access to bonus content, including detailed training plans, recovery tips, and more advanced techniques that will take your performance to the next level. Make sure to check it out for additional resources that are sure to help you stay at the top of your game!

For access to bonus content and resources, scan this QR Code or visit
https://theweekend-warrior.co.uk/warrior-resources

Chapter 2: Mindset – How to Win the Mind Game

"Our thoughts lead to emotion which leads to behaviour."

"How you think is how you feel, is how you behave."

In this chapter, I will discuss some psychological principles that I found helpful in a sporting context. Many of these have helped me personally and have been shown to help many highly successful teams and athletes, too. The power of the mind is vast; therefore, I will only scratch the surface of it and go through the principles that offer you the biggest wins in the shortest amount of time. I am not a psychologist, so all of these are how I understand and use the principles, as well as how others have used them successfully.

The Fight or Flight Response

Our body is controlled by our nervous systems; yes, did you know that a lot of people think we have just one nervous system? The truth is, we have several. I am going to describe some aspects of one of our nervous systems. I know it's odd, but stick with it.

As the name suggests, our Autonomic Nervous system is autonomic and generally works without our conscious control. It controls functions such as heart rate, breathing rate, blood pressure, body temperature, digestion, production of fluids, the balance of fluids, etc.

There exist two divisions of the autonomic nervous system: the sympathetic nervous system, also called 'fight or flight,' or the parasympathetic nervous system, called 'rest and digest".

So, we're either in 'fight or flight' or 'rest and digest' at any given time. Obviously, in modern society, we don't have to fight with people or run away very often, but what we do need to use our 'fight or flight' response for is when we are competing or exercising intensely. Why? Well, it allows us to access a system that can produce this highest level of physical and mental results. Our 'fight or flight' system helps us by increasing our breathing rate, heart rate, and blood pressure, all of which are natural reactions needed to produce significant physical or mental performance. This 'fight or flight' should happen only briefly, that is, when we need to it to perform well.

When we come out of 'fight or flight', we go into 'rest and digest'. Here, the opposite happens: our breathing rate goes down, blood pressure decreases, heart rate drops, and our bodies can repair naturally. We must be able to access this state to allow our bodies to focus on relaxing and repairing the structures that have been subject to increased stress.

What often happens is that we get into 'fight or flight' and we never actually come out of it again. That is a big problem for our health, both physically and mentally. Later down the line this can lead to many issues such as an increase in the risk of injuries, a plateau or drop in training improvements, and a lack of productivity which can be detrimental to our mental health and mindset. Overall, stress hormones continually increase in this state. It ultimately leads you to not think clearly, and as your behaviour is directly associated with your thoughts, your behaviours are consequently not clear and focused.

If you are stuck in 'fight or flight' longer than you should be, you will see several simple signs. For example, you'd find that you're struggling to sleep, feeling tired constantly, feeling tense, continually needing to go to the toilet, experiencing anxiety, experiencing an increased heart rate, and that you lack the ability to switch off.

It is therefore essential that we are able to access both 'fight or flight' and 'rest and digest' when needed, but it is equally crucial to move between these states in a controlled way.

As I mentioned, the autonomic nervous system is not consciously controlled. Still, there are things that we can do to encourage our bodies' unconscious control.

There are several things that you can do to help you get out of the constant state of 'fight or flight'. One of the easiest things to do is to use your breath. We can use the breath to consciously override that 'fight or flight' response. When you hyperventilate, for example – an extreme example of 'fight or flight' – breathing is very focused on the inhalation (breathing in) of air; we tend to inhale more often and for longer than we exhale (breathing out). We know that when we inhale, our breathing/heart rate goes up in 'fight or flight' response, and when we exhale it comes back down again. In this state, breathing techniques can play an incredibly important role in moving out of this state.

In the example above, we need to consciously focus on our breath, that is, try to expand the exhale for as long as possible. Doing so means that we can regulate the response in a controlled way.

Below a straightforward breathing exercise that can be done almost anywhere – it's a useful tool to keep in your back pocket when you want to move out of 'fight or flight'.

1. Slump down in your chair so that your shoulders are relaxed and your back is nice and relaxed (not having to work to keep you upright).
2. Slowly inhale through your nose for 4-6 seconds so the breath is almost silent.
3. Exhale for as long as you can, ideally you want to exhale for twice as long as you're breathing, approximately 8-10 seconds, again making sure the breath is almost silent.
4. Briefly pause before inhaling again.
5. Repeat

The first time you do this you may find it difficult to control your exhalation for twice as long. It is hard, but if you can get to that point it can have a real positive effect. Start with five minutes a couple of times a day and then gradually build it up as much as you can.

The Pygmalion Effect

The definition of the Pygmalion effect is one of two:

"An improvement in a person's performance when someone expects them to perform well or achieve more." [1]

"Occurs when an individual's behaviour conforms to their belief of how they are expected to behave, sometimes referred to as a self-fulfilling prophecy." [2]

The Pygmalion effect is a psychological principal we encounter very often in our daily lives. As with a lot of psychological principles, it is prevalent in a lot of things that we already do without knowing. When you understand it, however, you will be able to look back at times when you have used this principle for positive or adverse results. Bringing this principle to the conscious mind will allow you to use it more often and for the better.

This principle is very closely related to external and internal motivation. I will mainly discuss this from a sporting viewpoint, but this principle is prevalent in many other aspects of life such as school/university work, business success, DIY, etc.

---

[1] Rosenthal, R., & Jacobson, L. (1968). PYGMALION IN THE CLASSROOM: TEACHER EXPECTATION AND PUPILS' INTELLECTUAL DEVELOPMENT. New York: Holt, Rinehart & Winston

[2] Merton, R. K. (1948). THE SELF-FULFILLING PROPHECY. ANTIOCH REVIEW, 8(2), 193–210

In sport or professional roles, it's easy to perceive a message as an *expectation*. This is crucial to remember – if you hear it and believe it, it's more likely to happen. The Pygmalion principle has been proven to make that expectation more likely to happen. For example, if your coach strongly expects you to score a penalty, you will be more likely to score than if he/she didn't expect you to. Alternatively, if they don't expect you to be able to pick the right pass, then you are less likely to execute this.

As I have just described, expectations will significantly affect the result; therefore, it is important, where possible, to surround yourself with those positive environments and higher expectations in order to experience a positive outcome rather than a negative one. This is done by selecting the team you play for, the coaches you work with, and anyone else who interacts with you. Why? Because positive expectations effect performance.

Obviously, an external expectation is something that we can't always control. But don't worry: it doesn't mean that, if you experience negativity, then you are destined to fail. That is not the case. It does mean, however, that you need to be able to focus on your internal motivators and not let any of these external expectations change what your inner thoughts are saying.

As you now consciously understand that it is proven that expectations have a significant effect on the outcome, it will be easier for you to experience a positive impact.

To experience the highest benefit of this principle, it needs to be implemented. In other words, you need to believe it whole heartedly. Using the Pygmalion principle, it is crucial that we set our own expectations; we need to look for the positive outcome or achievement so as to make us more likely to achieve it. There are several ways you can start to implement this, and I will walk you through them in a straightforward way. It is simple and easily implemented, but to make it work it requires consistency and habit formation.

To start, you need to have an achievement in mind. Once you know what this is, you can then picture it happening. Remember, you need to make sure this image is very vivid; make sure you're in the picture. Keep this picture in your head until it feels like it is reality. It would help if you spent significant time picturing this image of you achieving this goal every day, and particularly as you get closer and closer to the actual achievement.

It is a very powerful technique despite it being so simple; it can also be implemented for any sort of goal. One level at which it may work is picturing winning the league with a certain team, or perhaps scoring over a certain amount of points. Alternatively, it could simply be the moment of scoring a goal or achieving a certain time at a running event. You can even practice this technique at a granular level – doing exercises at the gym, for example.

If you can't picture yourself doing it, the likelihood is that you will not be able to do it, even if your body is physically capable.

An example that I see a lot of in my private practice is when someone comes in with an injury. I ask, "what is your goal, or what do you aim to achieve after this injury is healed?" Unsurprisingly, a lot of people wish not to be in pain, but the truth is that that is not the real reason they came to see me. It can sometimes take someone a while to actually think about what their true aim is, whether that's playing a certain level of sport or winning a specific competition. Unless you have a particular goal pictured, you will not be efficient in your rehabilitation process.

The above misconception about the true nature of goals is a mistake that I have seen in the past, especially with long-term injuries in athletes who may never play again. The quicker the idea of failure gets turned into an image of achieving a goal, whatever that is, the quicker the athlete enjoys better focus and will both mentally and physically start the process of achieving his/her goal.

As I mentioned earlier, external factors can cause negative expectations and, therefore, negative outcomes. Luckily, the first step in mitigating this is knowing about it. Once you know it is happening, then you can do something about it. If you can't change the negative environment, it's not the end of the world: you just have to make sure *you* are controlled by your internal thoughts. If there is a negative comment or expectation from someone, you immediately picture yourself positively achieving that goal – the more vivid the picture, the better it will work. Once you get into the habit of doing this, the process will start to happen automatically and you'll begin forming a habit of positive expectation, thereby avoiding negative images occurring in the first place.

Did you know that the above is something that professional athletes have to do every single time they play? When you watch sports on TV you will often hear the phrase "his head has dropped," and without knowing it, the speaker is describing the exact negative expectation the player began believing about himself. When that player or athlete is playing in front of a crowd – whether that is five people or 50,000 – there is often negativity abound. If internalised, players may be badly affected. Obviously, the higher-pressure stages or larger audiences will require more conscious effort, but the general principle remains the same.

Does this also affect the referee to make biased decisions? I won't get into that one! ;)

It is not the Situation; It Is How You Handle It

Situations and events get blamed for a lot of negative thoughts and negative actions. But the truth is, many of these events are completely out of our control, yet we still blame them for causing stress or bad outcomes.

No one wants a negative outcome, but if something is completely out of your control, then dwelling on it is unproductive and will still not change the outcome. All this will cause a negative spiral of your thoughts that will result in you believing in negative expectations, thereby causing the effects I have just covered.

You cannot control every situation and its outcome, but you can manage your attitude towards it and how you deal with it. We all know that there are many factors in sports and in life that are entirely out of our control. For example, a wrong refereeing decision, a teammate's mistake, another team's result, an unavoidable injury, etc. We can't control these, especially when they have already happened, but there is something in all situations that we can control: how we react.

How we Think, Feel, and React

The reaction to any situation is crucial – both from a physical and mental perspective. We are always in complete control of our reactions, no matter what the situation is. As with anything that produces high rewards, it takes time and requires practice and commitment.

If a situation strikes us as bad, it will make us feel negative; we will then be more likely to react poorly. We need to change this cycle. Instead, we need to understand that the situation is something we can't control. Doing so means that we will feel motivated to do something we can control. In other words, we will react in a productive way. By changing this cycle, you can turn a negative situation into something that will ultimately benefit and motivate you to do something positive.

"We Didn't Fail… We Have Just Learnt Something That Doesn't Work."

A technique to help stay positive and change the cycle of negativity starts by asking yourself some simple questions:

Could I have controlled that outcome?

If *yes,* then analyse what you could have controlled using facts; this will give you something specific to improve. It means that when you next encounter that problem, you will be able to experience a better outcome.

If *no*, then go on to the next outcome, which you could control.

Could you have avoided the situation altogether?

If *yes*, work out what you could have done to avoid the whole situation then practice doing it.

If *no,* tell yourself there is nothing you could have done and then go on to the next outcome which you can control.

It is not quite as simple as asking two questions, both of which will – of course – not automatically solve all your negative thoughts immediately, but it is a start that will allow you to become more self-aware in situations that you have no control over. If you can master this then you will be able to let go of feelings of resentment and you'll be able to put your focus into something you can control.

How to Handle Pressure

One of the most important things you'll need to develop as an athlete is the ability to remain calm and perform well under pressure, even in the most chaotic of circumstances. A champion doesn't get flustered under pressure; they retain the ability to make good decisions, think clearly, and complete the task in front of them with confidence.

When performing under pressure, some athletes become smothered by it, whilst others beat the competition. Every athlete feels some pressure when performing, but the less prepared you are, the more you are going to feel. Pressure creates tension and can cause you to panic. Naturally, this is detrimental. The more you rush, the more mistakes you will make and the more pressure you will be under… which leads to more panic, more mistakes, and more pressure. You get into a negative spiral, which will cause performance to keep dropping.

Only a few people think about how they're going to handle high-pressure situations; most wait until it's too late. We have all heard of the term 'choke', that is, when someone's performance suffers greatly under pressure; their well-planned strategy crumbles and they fail to do things they have practised thousands of times in training. This is generally caused by a lack of confidence, negative opinions, or perceived results and not by your ability or skill set. If you can work out how to use pressure in a positive manner in order to aid your skill set, or to work out strategies to block out the negative external pressures, you will be able to avoid failure. You will perform the skills that you have honed over and over again, and you'll build your self-confidence.

Pressure isn't something that you should avoid. In fact, it is something you should use to your advantage. Whilst most people run from pressure, great champions learn to deal with it and use it.

Here are some strategies you can use to handle pressure and use it to your advantage:

Focus on the process and not the outcome. Avoid overthinking when under pressure by focusing on what you've trained to do. Concentrate on the process of a particular skill you have done repeatedly, and trust in your preparation. In training, ensure you have a specific process for the skill and repeat it as much as possible. Realise that all the hard work is already done, your training will pay off, and that it is time to enjoy performing in a competition.

Downplay the importance. The more important we believe an event to be, the more pressure we feel, so a brilliant way for people who feel a lot of pressure is to downplay the magnitude. It may feel counter-intuitive, but reducing the importance of an event can help take the pressure off. Try reframing the situation: think of an event as your opportunity to show yourself what you are truly made of and to perform at your best. You have nothing to lose: *you're either going to win or you're going to learn*. When you think like this, it can really help take the edge off of whatever pressure you're feeling. You came here to give it your best shot, so trust in your skills and go for it.

Breathe. When you're in a high-pressure situation, your breathing will likely become short and fast, something that will negatively affect your performance. To quickly reduce feelings of anxiety, focus on your breathing to depressurise the situation. It can help bring you back from panic to the present moment. Controlling and focusing on your breathing will distract you from the situation as well as get you out of the immediate 'fight or flight' response, as I mentioned earlier, thereby giving you clearer thinking.

Focus on what you can control. A lot of pressure comes from places that we cannot control. For example, an 80,000-person crowd watching you take a penalty. We cannot control this, and therefore we need to focus on something we can control – like our breathing or our process. Take yourself out of the pressure by controlling what you can – ignore trying to change what you can't.

You've earnt the right. The habit of confidence under pressure is learnt in training, that is, through your preparation. Remind yourself why you are in the situation. You have worked hard to improve your processes, skills, and fitness; you must remind yourself of the hard work that it's taken to get to where you are and remind yourself, too, that you have earnt the right to be there.

Pressure can be a positive, so find the balance. Pressure keeps you focused and keeps you sharp. If we feel too little pressure, we can lose focus and go just through the motions. Recognise that pressure can be positive if you are able to control it and use it to your advantage. You must accept that you will feel pressure during a performance and that it is normal to do so. Pressure is just your body telling you to wake up and pay attention; it is your body's way of getting you ready to perform. Take advantage of the pressure, get excited, and focus on what you want to happen... not what you're worried might happen.

Instant Versus Delayed Gratification

"Instant gratification is the desire to experience pleasure or fulfilment without delay or deferment." Putting it into easier terms, it is *getting what we want when we want it*. There's nothing wrong with wanting or needing things, experiences, or products in a timely manner, but it's important to balance our desires with a realistic sense of patience. By itself, though, instant gratification isn't a negative thing, yet when we expect instant results in everything we want to do, it becomes unrealistic and damaging.

When instant gratification becomes an uncontrollable expectation, you start to put the delayed effect or consequence to the back of your mind. It is then that you think about the immediate enjoyment or gratification rather than the impact down the line, the reality of which may be significantly worse. Here are some very common examples which may well be done without thinking of the consequences:

- Indulging in a chocolate bar that tastes fantastic at the time, but causes you to put on weight/fat later on.

- Hitting *snooze* instead of getting up early to exercise thereby missing out on those endorphins and likely resulting in not reaching the level of performance you would like to get to.

- Going out for drinks with your friends instead of finishing a paper or studying for an exam that you may fail.

- Going out for drinks with your friends instead of getting a good night's sleep on a work night or before a match, thereby reducing your performance significantly.

- Buying a new car that will require a high-interest loan instead of waiting until you have saved enough money to buy... leading you to pay double.

I'm not saying you shouldn't do any of these things, because of course it is important that you do enjoy life, but what I would encourage you to do is think of the second-order consequence of doing that thing, however big or small. The second-order consequence is the name for what happens down the road as a result. Similarly, you can think of the 3rd or 4th order consequence as longer-term effects.

If you want to compete at your highest potential, it is key to understand this principle not only in a sporting context, but in life.

This means thinking about the consequences of repeatedly eating a chocolate bar when you are hungry. If you do this, you're more likely to eat something healthy once you realise that the second-order consequence – a heavier weight – is a danger.

Usually, the things that you get instant gratification from are the things that cause adverse reactions in the long run. Alternatively, it is the times when we do something that will cause delayed gratification that we experience significant benefits.

"Delayed gratification refers to the ability to put off something fun or pleasurable now in order to gain something that is **MORE** fun, pleasurable, or rewarding later." To clarify, a significant ending to that definition is the MORE part. When there is delayed gratification, it is usually *more* rewarding than the gratification that you can get initially.

For many, it is getting increasingly harder to stay focused on delayed gratification rather than look at second-order consequences. The improvements in technology and infrastructure have resulted in the expectation that everything should happen instantly.

As an example, many people now use Amazon to order things that they want. The major appeal of Amazon is next-day – or even same-day delivery – in some places. This has now become the norm. A couple of years ago it would have taken at least a week to get anything online, yet now we can get almost anything within a day. This has caused many of us (me included) to buy things that we don't need just because of the ease of use and speed of the ordering process. If we had to make a special trip to a shop, or wait a while for something, we probably wouldn't bother.

Therefore, the second-order consequence is that we have a house full of things we don't need or use and have spent a load of money for the pleasure. To go further, the third-order consequence may be that we can't afford that big purchase of a house or holiday... because of years of small, instant parcels from Amazon!

The same applies to online streaming services. When I was younger, to watch a TV series you had to make sure you were sitting in front of the TV at a specific time. To watch a film, you had to have a day out at the cinema or go to the video store and rent one; you'd also have to take it back a few days later. Now, we have whole series' available at our fingertips – any time, day or night. All-in-all, we have come to expect instant gratification in everything we do.

Here are some tips to avoid getting stuck in the instant gratification frame of mind and to get to those significantly better results later down the line:

1. **Understand the principle.** Understanding what instant gratification means will bring about more awareness.
2. **Know what you want!** Get a sense of where you're going and what your target is. If you don't understand where you're going or what you are going to be working towards, then it's easy to get distracted by the temptations that life throws your way. Ask yourself: What do I want to achieve? When do I want to achieve this? How will I achieve this?
3. **Identify potential obstacles!** If you can predict things that might sidetrack you, then you can come up with a plan to deal

with them. You will also be able to see them coming. Ask yourself: What temptations could sidetrack me? How will I handle these temptations?
4. **Have a strong accountability network.** Having accountability is key to keeping you on track and having that support to avoid straying off the path is vital. It is always hard to stray off the path when you have someone else that you have told your goal to; he/she will be disappointed in you if you slip. This can be a friend, coach or anyone who will help to motivate you towards your goal. Ask yourself: Who could support me along this journey? How could they support me?
5. **Have a reward system.** Having small rewards along the way will give you short, medium, and long term things to look forward to. They will also stop you from getting sidetracked, especially if your goal is a long time away. It will be tough to delay all gratification for that long, so small excitements on the way will keep you on track.

That is how you can start working towards those higher levels of achievement by delaying gratification. As you can see, it all comes from knowing what your goal is then working backwards to get there – using the tactics above to stay on the path.

Sometimes we do get knocked off the path and into the instant gratification spiral. That is not a problem. Here are some tips on how to get back on track and towards your goals. The below are also helpful to think about for those smaller goals and temptations that may be causing adverse effects in your life.

1. **Ask yourself:** What will the consequences look like in 10 minutes? Ten days? Ten months? 10 Years? And if those consequences aren't significant, then you can carry on knowing that you are not going too far off the path. Alternatively, if they have significant consequences, then thinking of those consequences will show you that you are going to head significantly off the path. Then make a decision.
2. **Eliminate objects of temptation.** We don't often long for things that we don't think about. The best way to not think about

something is not seeing it. For Example, it's much easier to avoid junk food when it isn't in our homes.
3. **Monitor your distractions.** If we don't know what our bad habits are, then how can we change them? Phone, TV, and the internet are significant areas of instant gratification, thus it is very easy to get carried away with these and not realise how much time we are spending on them. All of these can be monitored so that we can set targets to reduce the amount over time.

Remember, though, you don't always need to say 'no' to things that make you feel good. Giving yourself a break once in a while is important, as is treating yourself to a reward after hard work. However, these occasional treats are much more valuable when you have made delayed gratification a habit.

Habits

All too often, we overvalue the implementation of a quick fix. We undervalue the impact of small decisions compounded on a daily basis. It is the minute decisions, when repeated and duplicated, that create unparalleled results and unexpected change.

Don't get me wrong, if we can get a result in a shorter amount of time then I am all for that, but often our expectations are not realistic.

"A habit is a settled or regular tendency or practice, especially one that is hard to give up." [3]

---

[3] **Oxford English Dictionary** (2020). Habit (2nd ed.). Oxford University Press

In other words, a habit is something that we repeatedly do. Habits can either be positive or negative, but understanding how habits have an exponential effect over time is essential. Using the techniques that I have mentioned previously, you can identify or create positive habits and expel negative ones. To understand how small habits have an exponential effect over time, you need to know about the *compound effect*.

The compound effect is the principle of doing a lot of small, seemingly insignificant actions performed repeatedly over a long period of time, thereby snowballing into incredible accomplishments.

It is often the case that a small action is quick and straightforward to do and a lot easier than a significant change. It is also easier to put off a big change. Therefore, it is often a lot easier to make a lot of small changes without too much effort and extra motivation. Of course, the opposite is true too – if you constantly repeat a negative action and thereby form a habit, the results will be equally negative. For example, having one more snack after dinner is fine, but if you compound that over a week, a month, a year, it adds up to a pretty poor diet that, if you really thought about it, you probably didn't need.

It's not our big choices, but the ones you think don't matter that derail you. So, the earlier you start making changes, the more the compound effect works in your favour.

Remember the following equation:

Small Choices + Consistency + Time = Significant Results

This chapter highlights one of the most crucial elements in your athletic journey: mastering the mental game. Your ability to control your mind, especially in high-pressure situations, is essential for peak performance. Understanding how to manage your autonomic nervous system shifting between 'fight or flight' and 'rest and digest' ensures both mental clarity and physical recovery. By leveraging psychological principles like the Pygmalion effect, you can set high expectations for yourself and meet them, ultimately driving your performance to new heights.

As we wrap up this chapter on mindset, remember that mental readiness lays the foundation for everything else. For more detailed strategies and tips on improving your mental game, scan the QR code provided.

For access to bonus content and resources, scan this QR Code or visit **https://theweekend-warrior.co.uk/warrior-resources**

Now, let's shift focus to another equally vital area, **time management**. Proper time management helps you balance your mental, physical, and life commitments to ensure you're on the path to success. Let's dive into how you can optimise your time to enhance performance.

Chapter 3: Time Management

Time is a precious commodity, and finding time to focus on sport can be tricky and can often be a barrier to achieving your goals or your actual potential. Being able to manage our time effectively and efficiently is a key skill, one which can often have the biggest impact on sporting performance. If you do not manage your time efficiently then you will not be able to implement any of the strategies in this book, and that will significantly reduce the likelihood of you achieving your goals.

There are very few people who can class themselves as professional athletes. Professional athletes – where their sport is their job – can prioritise their time and put the majority of their focus into improving their performance. I have been involved in professional sport for a while now, and behind the scenes of a professional athlete there is often a whole support team; they reduce the stress, plan the time, and give the athlete even more time to spend improving his/her performance. There is only a very small amount of people who get to this level.

Of course, it is hard when you juggle a full-time job around a sport you love, but it becomes even harder if you don't think about your time management. Some of the best uses of your time is to actually sit down and work out if you are managing your time well or if you are *busy being busy*. As such, I am going to go through some of the best ways in which you can learn to manage your time well, whether you are a professional, semi-pro, or amateur athlete juggling another job or a family. It doesn't matter what your current situation is, everyone will benefit from being more efficient with their time.

There are 168 hours in the week... this doesn't change. There are 24 hours in a day and 7 days in a week, which equates to 168 hours (24 hours x 7 days).

The average person sleeps for 8 hours per day equating to 56 hours a week. Let's assume our full-time job (with a commute) is 56 hours a week. We then need to account for general housework etc., which removes around 20 hours. This leaves us with 36 hours. Let's then take 10 hours for watching TV/playing games etc. That still leaves 26 hours a week to fill. So, the question is, is this time being spent achieving your goal, or is it being spent on procrastination?

Know Where You Are

One of the best places to start, at least from a time management point of view, is to know where you currently are. If you don't know where you currently are then how do you know if you are being efficient or not? So, right now, spend a whole week recording what you do: a basic 24 x 7 table with the days and the hours is just fine. It is important that you leave judgment words off so that it shows only what you've done during that time. For example, don't put down the word 'nothing' during the time you were chilling out over the weekend; write exactly what you were doing: sunbathing, watching tv, reading, or whatever the action was. It is also easier if you try and record the start and end times of the actions as you go along, rather than at the end of each day where your memory will limit you from being accurate.

This exercise alone can have a major benefit. It will increase your awareness and therefore start to help you to do things with more purpose. Being more aware of what you are doing is a very underrated action. You can use this for a lot more than increasing the awareness of your current time. In fact, you can use it to influence your future time.

There are a number of apps that you can use on your phone that will tell you how much time you spend on social media, on games, or just general procrastination. A lot of people will be surprised at how much time they spend on their phones each day; this usage has become a habit because of its accessibility. If you never track it, you will generally underestimate the amount of time you waste.

Does Your Time Reflect Your Priorities?

If the answer to this question is 'no' then you will reach your goal as quickly as you could do. If you know what your priorities are it is a brilliant start, but the next thing that we have to do is to make sure we are actually spending time on the important things. It might sound like a relatively simple thing to do, but it is very easy to become distracted – especially when it comes to instantly gratifying tasks.

To avoid getting side tracked and distracted from the goals, the real key is planning. Compartmentalising it is a really good way to be efficient and to reach a quality outcome. When you know where you are currently spending your time, then you need to start to look ahead and plan your day/week/month/year. How? Well, with specific blocks of time that you are going to spend on specific tasks. It is key that you have this written down so that when you look back at how you actually spent your time you can compare it with your plan.

When you have planned out these times for specific priorities it is crucial that you protect your time. Do not compromise.

Don't get too down-hearted if you look back and you don't manage to achieve the exact times spent on your tasks you set out with, however. It will take time and practice to work out how much time is needed on each type of task. The important thing is that you start doing it; make small improvements as you run into problems and make sure to allocate the appropriate time next time.

Be careful when setting your priorities. You have to be sensible when it comes to time frames. They have to be achievable, but challenging. There is a principle called *Parkinson's Law*. It that states "work expands so as to fill the time available for its completion".

This means that, if you set a timeframe that is too long you, you will just stretch that work over a longer period than is needed. Think back to school deadlines: whether the teacher set an assignment for tomorrow or next week, it would still get done, right? But, the longer you had, the more time you spent on it – and that extra time was probably spent on procrastinating.

Quantity And Quality Are Different Things

Just because you spend a long time doing something doesn't mean that it is quality work. We need to make sure that we spend time doing quality work and that we're not just busy being busy. You can spend as much time on something as you like, but it is completely pointless if it is not quality. For example, you could spend 5 hours a week practicing your penalties for years on end. On the surface you would think you must be brilliant and that you'll score every time, but actually, you've spent most of that time using the wrong foot or wearing a blindfold. The time spent is high, but the quality is very low. You would be better off spending significantly less time practicing if the practice sessions were of high quality.

In deliberate practice, you need to be fully focused on developing the skill you are working on whilst minimising distractions as much as possible. It has been shown that focusing intently takes so much energy that you can only sustain that level of practice for 60 to 90 minutes at a time. When you decide to improve one of your skills, keep this in mind – and have shorter but more deliberate practices.

It is important to consider the sport relative to your practice. If your sport is ultramarathon running, then cutting your runs short is not going to give you the endurance you need. You need to work out the requirements of your sport and then think about the time you'll spend practicing. Don't constantly do double the amount you think you need to. A football match is 90 minutes, so spending 3 hours on a training session every day is not relative to what is needed. You won't find an Olympic 100m sprinter doing 5km runs.

You may think professional athletes train for hours and hours, but in truth oftentimes training sessions are very short and sharp. They don't need to spend hours on the pitch if the quality of the session is high. If the outcome can be achieved in a shorter period of time, then the rest of the time spent is just wasted.

Even if you are doing an individual sport it is still crucial to protect you time. Anything that might distract you during that session should be avoided. Set time aside before or after your session to do things that will distract you or reduce the quality of your session. If you go to a public gym and you know there is always someone in there that has a chat mid-way through your routine, go 10 mins earlier and chat with that person first. In this way, when you start training you are completely focused on it.

Multitasking is Overrated

Multitasking is overrated. The science is clear: the best way to do a poor job of a task is to do it alongside another task. The more engaged or focused with a particular task we are, the higher the quality will be. The more you try to do at once, the worse the outcome will be. You should only have 1-3 priorities at a time; any more and you will start to lose clarity. More than a couple of priorities will cause you to take longer to achieve them, or you may achieve them to a lower quality than what you are capable of.

Prioritise your tasks. Have them written down and cross them off when you have achieved them. You need to spend time thinking about what these priorities are, and how they are ordered, so as to have clarity about the path you need to take. Doing this will mean that you can analyse your performance and therefore tweak your plan as needed.

When you know what your priorities are you can start to work on one task at one particular time. If you are trying to develop a particular skill, then make sure that time is specifically dedicated to that one aspect and not to developing 10 skills at one time. Doing so means that yes, you can develop the other skills, but you're dedicating quality time to each; doing this means you can skilfully switch between them at any given time.

The All Blacks Rugby Team are renowned for being an incredibly clinical team. They focus the majority of their time on basic skills. Until they have mastered those they will not go into a situation where they are expected to do a skill under pressure, especially if they can't do it under low pressure circumstances. Change your mindset.

Being Accountable

Accountability in sport is doing what you say you're going to do in a timely fashion and then executing the task to the best of your ability. But it also means being able to put your hand up and say 'this is what I need to do better or different'. Being accountable is not making excuses, not blaming others, or complaining. Accountability in sport is taking ownership of something and making sure you 'know your job and do your job' 100% of the time.

It is always easier to be accountable to other people than ourselves. If all we ever do is let ourselves down then it can be very easy to brush off. If you are accountable to someone else, whether that is a team, a coach, a company, etc. then it is a lot harder to let them down. It can be as simple as telling your friends or your family what your goals are and when you are going to achieve them.

A different way of doing it is bringing someone else in on your goals and working on them as a collective. For example, practicing your goal kicking with a team-mate in rugby union. You both commit to staying for half an hour after training to practice kicking; you take it in turns to stand behind the posts and collect the balls. If one of you doesn't turn up for the session, then you are causing your team mate to have to work twice as hard by having to collect the balls after each attempt. It is harder to let someone else down than it is to let yourself down. If you are an individual athlete, try and have a training partner or a coach who you train with in exactly the same way.

When I played rugby in the middle of winter – in knee deep mud – it would have been very easy to look out the window and stay in bed, but I always went because I didn't want to let my team mates down.

Make Use of Travel Time

We are spending a lot more time traveling, whether that is commuting to work or to training. This time is often spent by just listening to the radio or music; it is generally just being written off as wasted time, but it doesn't have to be. In fact, it can be a great way to find an extra hour or two a day. If you are looking to be more efficient with your time, then using this travel time for something productive is a very simple way.

If you are driving, then you are quite restricted: there are lots of podcasts or audio books that you can listen to whilst driving, however, many of which focus on specific skills and goals.

If you are traveling by train, coach, or plane then you have a lot more freedom. Why not do some video analysis of your performance, plan your schedule, watch a webinar on a particular skill or coaching style, or write?

Pass on Low Outcome Tasks

Low outcome work does not reflect your priorities, and therefore it takes you off of the path.

An analogy that I have found helpful is washing the car. I will be completely honest... I don't wash my own car; I pay someone to do it for me. The way that I see this is not as a luxury, but as prioritising my time. I could wash my own car, but it would take me over an hour to do and by the time I've got everything out and put everything away, I've lost all that time. Instead, I drop off my car on my way to work. This process takes a maximum of 5 minutes. For me this saves me the best part of an hour.

If I spend my time well, the money that I can earn in that hour is a lot more than what was spent to take the task off of my hands. So, what may sound like a luxury actually means that I can make money. This is an obvious business example, but it is exactly the same in a sporting context. The hour that you spend washing the car could be spent training, thereby improving your performance and getting closer to your goal. In this situation, you have to work out whether paying money to be able to spend more time training is worth it.

Everyone's circumstances are different, so I'm not saying never wash your car – you just have to work out if there are things you can avoid or delegate in order to prioritise your time.

Another point I need to mention is that if a task is something that you enjoy doing and it comes out of your relaxation or enjoyment time, then there is no problem in doing it. For me, some DIY, like putting up a shelf or fixing a door, is something that I strangely enjoy, so I will watch less TV or read less in that week and relax/recover by doing some sort of DIY. Crucially, though, that time does not come out of my prioritised time – it comes out of my relaxing time.

This only works with things that actually need to be done, not things that you are using as an excuse to be distracted. Do you really need to rearrange those ornaments on the mantel piece for the fifth time this month, or are you just telling yourself it is a must-do task because you don't what to do something else that is hard or uninteresting, despite the fact that it would get you closer to your goal?

I have 2 questions on my office wall; both remind me of my time management and stop me from getting side-tracked. In fact, staring at these all day, every day, is one of the reasons I have been able to prioritise my time and get this book written!

1. "Is this the best use of your time?"

2. "Does today's schedule reflect your priorities?"

These two questions are two of the ways I use to keep me on track and onwards towards my goals, whatever they may be at that time. The first one makes me think about what I am currently doing, that is, have I gotten distracted by something? The second question reminds me that I need to know what my 2 current priorities are and that I need to make sure I have planned to get them done no matter how tedious they may seem.

I am not saying that you should take out every bit of wasted time. We all need a break to give our bodies and minds a chance to recover. It is important to relax and do things that we love to do, even though they don't directly work towards our goals. But, it is crucial that you don't do too much of this and spend too much time on things that take you further away from achieving your goals.

Plan Time to Recharge/Recover

I have spoken a lot about planning your time around your priorities – which can often mean spending time on physically or mentally taxing tasks. These are obviously directly related to your goals, but you also need to make sure you are putting in blocks of time where you let your body or mind have a break. If you try to be focused 24-7, then you will very quickly burn out and your body will crash. Some signs of this type of breakdown may be that the quality of your work decreases, whether that be in physical markers or mental agility.

Make sure you plan time to do things you enjoy, like watching tv or playing computer games. It may sound like I am going back on a lot of what I have just said, but taking breaks means that, when you go back to your tasks, you will be physically and/or mentally recharged, thereby allowing you to spend the set time doing quality work and not working yourself into the ground. It is important that these times are planned in, just not too often. It calls for a fine balance which will take a bit of trial and error; everyone will need different amounts of recharging depending on how they function and what the actual tasks they are doing are.

Ultimately, it goes back to knowing where you are spending your time and how you are planning the future. If you find that the previous week, month or year you got burnt out, then you can plan for more recharging. Make sure you put this in with your competition schedule, so you know when you need to be fresh, or you know when you may be likely to burn out.

Learn to Say No

If you keep adding things to your list, you will dilute your priorities. Say 'no' to things that are going to get in the way of your goals. I am not saying never do anyone any favours, but you do need to make sure that you don't constantly push your priorities down the line for something that isn't part of your goals. Be transparent with your priorities, and often, if others know that you are working hard towards a target, they will only ask you for help if it is important or if it will help both of you. If someone doesn't know that you are training hard for a marathon, then they may ask you if you can spend a few days helping move house. Whereas, if they know what you are doing then they wouldn't ask you or they would do so only after the event. If someone doesn't know that you are working hard towards a goal then just tell them that you are and that you can't help until you have achieved it, or if you really do want to help sooner then you can use some of your relaxation time to do it rather than taking away your protected time.

Know When to Finish

Sometimes we need to know when to simply finish a session early or miss one altogether. No matter how much planning we do... things happen. For example, people may have a bad night's sleep or are overtrained mentally or physically. When this happens, it can be more valuable to just call it a day early rather than continuing with a bad session. As I mentioned earlier, quality is so important: if for whatever reason the quality is so low that it's going to be difficult to raise it, then carrying on the session will only cause poor outcomes and for you to become angry or annoyed with your practice – this is quantity over quality.

This should be done objectively rather than emotionally. For example, if a runner feels like a session isn't going well, but their timings say differently, then they certainly shouldn't stop. In contrast, if they are 30% slower than normal and feeling like it is not going well, then stopping would avoid the athlete going into a negative spiral. It is worth having objective markers on the performance at training, and if those numbers are significantly worse during one normal training session, then an assessment can be made.

The psychology pointers from chapter 2, and the time management ones from this chapter, will give you the keys to the rest of this book. I recommend that you re-read both chapters again just to make sure you are building strong foundations before moving on to the rest of the book. These are proven strategies that are timeless and will always be worth going back through at any point, particularly if you are starting to drift off the path you want to head down.

We will now head into a series of chapters which are focused on your activities, sports, and keeping you on track. There are loads of practical tips and tricks coming up, all of which you can implement for preventing, treating and rehabbing injuries as well as training and recovery in general.

Don't forget, you can find more information on all of the strategies in this book. For access to bonus content and resources, scan this QR Code or visit **https://theweekend-warrior.co.uk/warrior-resources**

Chapter 4: Injury Prevention

"Injuries are the biggest reason that stop people taking part in sport or cause people to change the sport they love."

This statement is the best reason that you can have to try and avoid injuries and thereby keep doing the sport you love.

It is Impossible to Prevent all Injuries

Injuries are a part of sport and exercise; when you put your body under stress it is inevitable that there will be times during which certain structures are pushed too hard issues and damage occurs. Not all injuries are within our control. They can be caused by external sources, too. For example, in team sports you have several other people on the pitch whose movements and actions you cannot control. Even if you take part in an individual sport there are external factors such as equipment, weather, surfaces and other people which can all cause an injury.

Therefore, preventing all injuries is not realistic. It has also been shown that we cannot predict injuries or when they will happen. We can, however, reduce the risk of getting injured in the first place.

In a general sense, this involves improving strength, stability, and proprioception (balance) of specific structures, which will allow your body to be more robust; it will be able to cope with the stress that you put it under during sport as well as the unexpected stress and forces that you cannot control. For example, a late/high tackle in rugby, a studs-up slide tackle in football, or an unexpected pot-hole when running.

This involves a different approach to your normal training and it will be specific to your sport. It is also different to your gym/strength training. An extra session should be added to your training plan with the sole aim of injury prevention; it can be added before your gym/strength session or sports-specific training.

The training that you will do for your specific sport, as well as your strength training, will help prevent injuries. Being fit, strong and technically good at your sport will help in reducing injuries, too, but on its own it is not good enough to prevent injuries to the level which we should strive for. Remember, if you are injured, you are not able to do your sport. Therefore, there should be a massive emphasis on doing as much as you can to prevent problems that will stop you from doing your sport.

The Requirement of the Sport

The sport or exercise that you do puts specific demands on the body and will be vastly different depending on which sport it is. It is crucial that you know what these demands are, because if you *don't* how do you know what it is you need to train the body to withstand? It's also worth pointing out that the demands of your sport will be different at the different level you compete at. For example, for football the demands on the running load will differ significantly for the Premiership than loads in smaller competitions. It is important that you not only look at the demands of the sport, but the demands at the level in which you compete at or are aiming to compete in.

If in doubt you should always look at the demands of the sport at a level above you, as this will give you a buffer for when you improve. There is no harm in trying to set yourself up to be a more robust athlete than you are currently.

The demands required for sports are constantly changing depending on rule changes, techniques, players improving, surfaces changing, etc. Therefore, I will not be outlining any specific demands related any sports in this book other than for use as examples. All of the examples I use are correct at the time of writing this book, but may not be the case when you read this.

There are many ways to find the demands of your specific sport at different levels. There is a lot of data on elite sport, especially as more technology becomes available. In professional rugby, the players I work with wear GPS monitors which gives us information such as meters run, speed, meters in different speed zones, etc. They also wear heart rate monitors. All of this data is analysed to work out the general requirements of specific positions. This data also allows us to work out what the players need to do at the weekend. This data is very specific to our team and our sport, but there are a lot of studies that have got data from a number of teams and documented the average requirements of the sport at these levels. This is the same for a lot of higher-end team sports. To find this data for yourself, simply search for journal articles from the last 5 years on Google Scholar: 'the requirements of {insert your sport]'. If this data isn't available for your sport, then you will have to dig a bit deeper into sport science books related to that sport.

There may not be data on all sports and at all levels in published literature, but don't panic. It is possible to work a lot of the requirements out yourself without the need for any fancy technology. Start with breaking down your sport into its different components. This is a lot easier for sports which have fewer external components, such as cycling. You can start with a pen and paper and write down what an event looks like for you; for example, a football match requires me to play for a certain number of minutes and within that time do I take a certain amount of shots/passes/side steps, etc. The more depth that you go into, the better. Take your time working this out.

What if I do More than One Sport?

That is no problem at all, although it will require a little more work; you'll simply need to look at the requirements of all of the sports, as above, and then put them together to work out the requirements as a whole.

This is where it changes slightly from the requirements of the sports to the *requirement of what I want to be able to do*. This is crucial if you want to avoid over training.

For example, you may play football for a Sunday League team and be a CrossFit athlete, too. You would start by looking at the requirements of both individually, as I mentioned above. Then you need to look at your individual requirements: you need to look at what the scheduled sessions are for each sport. It may look like this:

Day	Scheduled CrossFit Training	Scheduled Football Training
Monday	Training	
Tuesday	Training	
Wednesday		Training
Thursday	Training	
Friday		
Saturday	Competition	
Sunday		Match

From this very simple starting point you are then able to build out the requirements during a normal week. In this example, you need to be able to cope with three CrossFit training sessions, a competition, one football training session, and a match each week.

If you followed step one, you will have looked into what the requirements of each session would be, then you'd have added it together and seen the week as a whole. From this data we can now understand what the body is going to be put through and be able to cope with. You have looked at the requirements of the sports individually then put them together to see a whole picture.

When you do this for yourself you need to plan as far ahead as you can, because not only do you need to understand what your body goes through in a week, but also how long it will go on for: how long the season is, the breaks, and the competitions or matches that are most important to you.

When you can plan in this way you may find that the amount of activity you would like to do is not realistic. Knowing this will allow you to change the expectation and will avoid burn out. I speak more about this in the training methods chapter later on.

Know the common injuries associated with your sport. Do some research into the most common injuries in your sport; this data is well documented. If we know the injures that happen frequently, then we can work to reduce the risk via our injury prevention program. For example, one of the common injuries in grassroots football (at the time of writing this) is ankle sprains. Knowing this means we can spend a significant amount of effort in our prevention program on the ankle and not, for example, the wrist.

Screening

Screening – sometimes you'll hear it called medical screening or a medical – specifically for sports and activity is a process used to evaluate a person's physical health and fitness before participating in sports activities.

This screening typically includes a comprehensive assessment of medical history, a physical examination, and, sometimes, additional tests like cardiovascular evaluations or musculoskeletal assessments. The primary goal is to identify any potential health risks that could compromise safety during activity. Early identification of such risks helps prevent injuries, improve performance, and ensure fitness for participation in a chosen sport or activity.

Firstly, if you have skipped step one of understanding the requirements of the sport then this part will be difficult. It is not to say that it can't be done, but the screen will be generic and generalised.

There is no set of screening tests that is best to do. They are specific for your sport, so I will therefore offer some common examples used across multiple sports. Remember, you need to refer to the requirements of your specific sport to make these most relevant to you.

The model I use for screening can be split into two components, the first of which is *strength and conditioning* screening. The second is *medical* screening.

Strength and conditioning screening has the aim of testing the fitness and strength of an athlete, as well as his/her physical attributes. This is generally for performance. These tests include gym-based exercise such as monitoring maximum weight resistance. Fitness is tested by using tests such as a 40-metre sprint, a 5km run, the bleep test, a 505-agility test, a max bike output, etc.

Next is the physical screening. This includes things such as the measurement of body fat, weight, height, etc. and can go as far as blood tests to assess nutritional deficiencies. I have outlined a few tests below, but to reiterate, they need to be specific to your sport. If you are a 100m sprinter, then doing a 10km run or agility drill as a screening test would not be as relevant as a 40m sprint.

Medical Screening uses the same principals as strength and conditioning tests, but instead of looking at overall strengths or fitness, more specific imbalances and stability issues are analysed. There is a significant crossover between the two. Included in medical screening is, as the name suggests, medical condition analysis. This includes things such as heart problems, diabetes, allergies, etc. which are crucial to know about and to avoid any serious problems.

Of course, many medical conditions will already be known about – for example, cardiac screening is a requirement for all professional athletes on a yearly basis. Cholesterol and diabetic checks should also be done regularly.

Medical screening can then be broken down further into tests for range of movement, strength, capacity, and movement patterns. This part of the screening should directly reflect the common injuries related to your sport in order to identify risks that could make you more likely to experience them. Range of movement testing, for example, may involve a knee-to-wall test for ankle range, or a straight leg raise for hamstring flexibility. Strength tests, from a medical screening perspective, are used to find imbalances. These tests may include single leg squats, calf raises, knee extensions, shoulder rotations, or hip strength tests. When it comes to capacity tests, repeated movements such as calf raises, side plank, hamstring bridges, etc. may be used to analyse endurance and capacity.

Finally, we move on to movement patterns; these are harder to quantify, but they are arguably the most important in order to observe inefficient movements or the inability to maintain stability. It is often useful to film these movements, after which they can be analysed more effectively. Movements may include single leg squats or single leg jumps, for example. There are scoring systems for looking at movement patterns,: the landing error scoring system (LESS) for landing errors is one example.

It might sound like a lot of tests and exercises, but remember to pick only the relevant ones for your particular sport.

In professional sport it is often the case that the first week of pre-season is solely dedicated to screening and testing.

A list of these tests that I have used can be found in the bonus content available via scanning the QR code, or simply visit
https://theweekend-warrior.co.uk/warrior-resources

Program Building

Now that we have the information we need, we can start putting a plan together. You should now be able to identify some areas in which you need to work. We can now pick specific exercises that will help you improve in these areas.

To do this you will need to be as specific as possible, and you'll need to be as targeted as you can. Pick exercises that can be done with limited equipment and effort, as this makes it easier to stick to and to do anywhere.

The exercises should not be too taxing or too hard. We will also be doing them before your normal training, so you do not want to fatigue. You don't need to use heavy weights, either; bodyweight is often enough. Depending on the time you have available, I would recommend up to 6-8 exercises in one session.

Do the exercises around 3 -4 times a week in order to get the best effect. You should do these exercises before you do your normal training session to prepare for the upcoming stress on the body. It is important that these form part of a separate session before your warm-up – they are not just replacing your warm-up. Warm-ups will be discussed in the 'training methods' chapter.

It should only take you about 15-20 minutes to get through everything. If you do take longer than this, you will start to move into a training session rather than injury prevention. On your rest days it doesn't matter as much, just that you do get the exercises done.

Technique

Technique is important in most areas, but especially when doing our prevention exercises. As discussed previously, we are doing these exercises because our bodies have weaknesses or poor movement patterns, so if we don't have a technique that is spot-on, then our bodies will do what they does best that is, compensate. Essentially, this will cause us experience the opposite of what we are aim for.

So, spend the time getting your techniques perfected with every exercise, no matter what it is. I t is important to keep re-checking your technique, as it can be easy to slide back into bad habits after a while, particularly if you get distracted. If you are not sure whether you're doing the technique correctly, then you can film yourself and look back at the footage; you can even send it to a qualified person to review it.

Exercises focussing on technique should be challenging in some way – whether that is balance, strength, or stability – but you should still be able to do them. It may take a while to get the technique perfect, so make sure you practice and regress the intensity when needed.

Compliance

As mentioned in the mindset chapter, the importance of the compound effect is equally as fitting here. Exercises which are in your injury prevention program may not be the most exciting of exercises – you may not be lifting as much as you can or going as fast as you can; you're doing small bodyweight or light exercise and it may therefore be hard to motivate yourself to do them. You won't see the direct results that you're used to seeing, but If you can make it a habit and avoid injuries then it will have a much bigger effect down the line. This is a perfect example of delayed gratification in sport. Remember, 15 minutes, 3-4 times a week, is all it takes to significantly reduce the risk of injury, all so that you can keep doing your sport!

Re-Test

How do we know If our injury prevention strategy is working?

There are two ways. The first is by asking yourself whether you have an injury. If you have recently had an injury, then your injury prevention isn't working or you haven't been doing it for long enough. You could also have been unlucky in that the injury you have wouldn't have been prevented because the forces were too big. In other words, it was one of the injuries that I spoke about earlier in the chapter and just impossible to prevent.

The second way to see if your prevention program is working is the more preferable way: re-test. The tests you did in the screening – before you started the program – should be repeated. The data you have from the first time you did your screening program is your base line, that is, your starting point. As such, the screening tests needs to be re-done in the same way in which they were originally done. As I explained earlier, the protocol for these tests needs to be comprehensive. So, when you do the re-test make sure nothing has changed; that way, the data used for comparison is as arcuate as possible.

Once the re-test has been done you need to look at the data: put it into a spreadsheet next to the base line data. You can then plot this into a graph and can therefore see it visually. You'll be able to see how far away you are from your goal.

When you compare the baseline and your re-test, you need to analyse it. If you have improved on a specific test, then your intervention is working and you should carry on. If your re-test hasn't improved, or even worse, has decreased, then you need delve into this in more detail.

- There are a few questions which you need to answer:
- Was your testing protocol the same as the screening?
- Were you fatigued when you re-tested?
- Have you been doing the exercises?
- Have you been using the correct techniques?
- Have you been doing the program for long enough?

If the answer to any of these questions is 'yes' then the exercises you were doing are not working and you will need to change them. G back to the program building phase for the specific exercises. Look at the screening test and analyse which muscles are involved in this movement. Then, look at exercises in the way mentioned previously and pick an exercise that will target this specific muscle. One done, decide on the frequency and load. Finally, do it... and do it consistently.

How often should you re-test your screening?

There are a couple factors which will determine how often you should re-test your screening data.

Firstly, as mentioned before, you need to do your screening when your body is rested. A re-test in a high intensity period of the season will not provide reliable results.

Secondly, if in your initial screening you find that your numbers are significantly above what's required then it is not particularly important to re-test these often. If you find that a number is significantly below the target, however, then it poses a significant risk and it therefore needs to be looked at more often.

Taking the above into account, you have to decide on the frequency of re-tests, whether that be every 2 weeks or more. Why? Because you are unique and you need to plan accordingly.

It is important to note that the re-test does not have to be every test, every time. If the majority of your tests are around the target, yet there are 3 that are significantly below, I would recommended that you just test the 3 putting you at the most risk. Test these every 2 weeks and then do the whole battery of tests every 6-8 weeks.

Cross Training

The definition of cross training is: "the action or practice of engaging in two or more sports or types of exercise in order to improve fitness or performance in one's main sport."

Cross training involves doing activities that are not a part of your specific sport. Most training programs involve some form of cross training, for example a runner may do a session on a bike or in the pool, a rugby player doing a gym session, or a tennis player playing football.

Cross training can be useful in several ways, the first being that it can provide a break from the normal stress of training in your sport, therefore allowing muscles, tendons, bones, joints, and ligaments a break. I will speak more about this in the recovery methods chapter.

Cross training is also a great way to condition different muscle groups, develop a new set of skills, and challenge the body after hitting a plateau. A plateau is reached when there is no apparent improvement in performance, even though the intensity of the practice remains the same. This usually happens after a long time spent doing the same exercises; this causes the body to be extremely efficient at performing those movements, thereby stopping progression to the next level. Furthermore, cross training allows you to vary the stress placed on specific structures such as muscles, tendons, ligaments, and joints. This will allow you to get over that plateau, as your body won't get used to being stressed in the same way each month. The structures will be constantly challenged in different ways which therefore causes the body to be more robust in a higher variety of situations.

In addition to the above, cross training will help you avoid over-training or overuse injuries whilst still allowing you to train. Therefore, you'll be able to fit more training into your schedule and use your time more efficiently. For example, if you try to improve your aerobic fitness as a runner, then you can do sessions in the pool or on a bike - these will improve your overall aerobic fitness which, in turn, will improve your running all without the repeated impact. This will allow you to add extra training sessions to your plan without the risk of overuse.

Cross training also helps to reduce muscle or movement imbalances in the body, all of which place you at risk of injuries. A lot of sports cause imbalances, as they require you to us specific parts of the body more than others. This will often result in either overuse or neglect in the areas that you don't use as much, thereby increasing the risk of injury. For example, if you are a right winger in rugby, you will often sidestep off of your right foot, so will tend to train that movement a lot more. Doing so neglects stepping off of your left foot. Thus, the odd time that you have to step off of your left side, your body will not be as robust in that movement and you may be injured or underperform. More obvious examples are in sports which require equipment use on one side, such as golf, tennis, canoeing, etc. These movements will cause significant imbalances to one side if left unaddressed. After some time, your injury risk will increase.

A tennis player may develop muscle imbalances in the dominant side of his body, especially in the shoulder of the serving arm. Thousands of serves over a season will cause the muscles in the playing arm to become significantly stronger whilst the other side's muscles will become weaker. In this instance, cross training will help to achieve balanced strength and stability in both the dominant and non-dominant sides. This balancing of strength and mobility helps to prevent one muscle group from pulling the body out of natural alignment. It can also prevent muscle tears caused by one muscle exerting more force than the other side can counter.

Cross Training for Kids

There is a longstanding debate in sport as to whether children should be encouraged to specialise in a particular sport at a young age or not. So, if your child wants to become a footballer then should every physical activity involve football? I am not going to get involved with this from a performance point of view, but from an injury prevention one there are a significant amount of studies out there that have proven the following: children are at a 30% higher risk of injury playing only one sport than if they take part in a number of sports. [4]

A common fear among parents is that, if their children don't play more and more of their specific sport, they'll fall behind and won't be as good of an athlete. It may actually be the opposite, however.

---

[4] Alison E. Field, Frances A. Tepolt, Daniel S. Yang, Mininder S. Kocher. **Injury Risk Associated With Sports Specialization and Activity Volume in Youth**. *Orthopaedic Journal of Sports Medicine*, 2019; 7 (9): 232596711987012

If children do too much of a specific sport, they may get injured and fall behind because they have to take time out from sport altogether.

Interestingly, cross training has significant effects on reducing the injury risk, particularly when it comes to children. So, it is important that a multitude of sports are practiced, but the overall load must be kept at a sensible level.

How to Cross Train

Most training programs already include some form of cross training. When you are designing your training plan you need to plan for a session that is not involved with your sport. Any exercise or activity can be used for cross training if it is not a skill associated with your particular sport. Weight training is a commonly used cross training tool. Other activities include swimming, cycling and running.

There is no one-size-fits-all when it comes to cross training, so you have to plan it around your own sport. Aim to make about 40% of your sessions centred around an activity other than your sport. Break down your sport into its base physiological components so that the cross training itself will help towards the demands of your sport. For example, if lower body strength is required then using weights as part of your cross training is relevant, or if your sport requires aerobic endurance then a long cycle or swim will help.

3d Printed Orthotics

"Your bed and your shoes. if you're not in one you're in the other"

Orthotics are medical devices used to modify the structural and functional characteristics of the neuromuscular and skeletal system, starting at your feet - your foundations. 3D printing technology now allows for the creation of orthotics that are perfectly contoured to fit the unique shape of each individual foot. This bespoke design approach facilitates better distribution of weight and balance, which is crucial in preventing overuse injuries or the worsening of existing conditions.

We now know that the prevention of injuries is paramount, and 3D-printed orthotics play a pivotal role in this. Athletes, particularly those in high-impact sports like running, benefit from using these custom-made devices. They help in aligning joints and reducing undue stress on specific areas such as the ankles, knees, and hips. For instance, a study published in the *Journal of Sports Science* highlighted that athletes using 3D printed insoles experienced a significant reduction in the incidence of stress fractures and other repetitive strain injuries.

Injury prevention extends beyond sports. Daily activities such as walking, climbing stairs, or prolonged standing can lead to discomfort and injuries over time. 3D printed orthotics help in maintaining proper foot alignment, which can prevent conditions like plantar fasciitis, bunion development, and joint pains. This proactive approach in daily life settings underscores the importance of 3D technology in enhancing overall musculoskeletal health.

The custom nature of these prints allows you to mitigate variations in shoes. Having a custom insole allows you to move it from shoe to shoe, which causes your foot to feel the same and, more importantly, have the same level of support that you have been diagnosed to need in every shoe you use. This includes most types of athletic footwear, including running shoes, walking shoes, cycling shoes, walking shoes, ski boots, football boots, etc. Nowadays, there are so many different types of shoes... and for each type, there are hundreds of brands with thousands of models. Using your custom orthotic is therefore a game-changer when it comes to footwear. When you have been prescribed your custom orthotic, you have the freedom to choose any footwear without having to compromise and risk injury.

Recovery from musculoskeletal injuries often involves the use of orthotics to stabilise and relieve pressure from the injured area. 3D printed orthotics offer a significant advantage here due to their custom-fit nature. They can be designed to accommodate swelling, support specific parts of the body, and adjust to changing rehabilitation needs, all of which can accelerate the healing process.

Clinical research shows that patients recovering from surgeries, such as ACL reconstruction or Achilles tendon repairs, benefit markedly from 3D printed orthotics. These devices are tailored to the specific stages of a patient's recovery, allowing for adjustments in the level of support and flexibility needed at each phase. It is well published that people experience shorter recovery times and improved outcomes when incorporating custom orthotics into treatment plans.

At my clinics, we often integrate 3D printed orthotics into rehabilitation programs. These orthotics aid in the correct redistribution of weight and the proper alignment of the body, both of which are essential for effective rehabilitation. In addition, the ability to frequently update the orthotic design to respond to a patient's evolving needs is a game-changer in rehabilitating from injuries.

The comfort provided by 3D printed orthotics is rooted in their ergonomic design. By aligning with the natural contours of the foot and the biomechanics of the body, these orthotics reduce pressure points, enhance stability, and decrease the overall discomfort associated with many foot ailments.

The future of 3D printed orthotics looks exciting and promises to be packed with continuous innovations in the field. Advancements in 3D printing materials, such as the development of more flexible, durable, and lightweight composites, are expected to further enhance comfort and functionality. Additionally, the integration of smart technologies, such as sensors to monitor stress and load, will provide real-time feedback, thereby allowing for dynamic adjustments to the orthotic's design.

Scan this QR code for more information on the 3d printed orthotics I recommend. I am currently wearing a pair while writing this at my standing desk and I would not be without them!

Orthopaedic Pillows and Mattresses

Orthopaedic bedding is specifically designed to support the body's musculoskeletal system. Unlike conventional pillows and mattresses, orthopaedic variants provide targeted support to ensure proper alignment of the spine and joints. This alignment is crucial in preventing stress and strain on the body, which can lead to chronic pain and injuries over time.

Orthopaedic pillows, for instance, are contoured to support the natural curve of the neck and head. They help maintain the spine's alignment, reducing the likelihood of waking up with a stiff neck or headaches. Similarly, orthopaedic mattresses are engineered to support the spine's natural curvature and distribute body weight evenly, preventing pressure points that can lead to discomfort and injuries.

The effectiveness of orthopaedic pillows and mattresses lies in their design and the materials used. These products are often made from high-density memory foam, latex, or hybrid materials that combine the benefits of both. Memory foam, in particular, is known for its ability to conform to the body's shape, providing personalised support and reducing the risk of pressure-related injuries.

Memory foam pillows and mattresses respond to heat and pressure, moulding to the body's contours and providing support where it is needed most. This support helps maintain proper spinal alignment, which is crucial for preventing injuries. When the spine is correctly aligned, there is less stress on the muscles, ligaments, and discs, thereby reducing the risk of strains and sprains.

Latex, on the other hand, offers a firmer support, yet one that is still responsive to the body's movements. It is naturally hypoallergenic and resistant to dust mites, making it an excellent choice for individuals with allergies or respiratory issues. Latex mattresses provide a balanced combination of support and comfort, ensuring that the body is well-supported without feeling overly rigid.

One of the most common areas of concern when it comes to sleep-related injuries is the back and neck. Poor sleeping posture can lead to chronic back pain, herniated discs, and other spinal issues. An orthopaedic mattress and pillow can significantly reduce the risk of these problems by providing the necessary support to maintain the spine's natural alignment.

Back injuries often result from poor posture and inadequate support while sleeping. When the spine is not properly aligned, the muscles and ligaments in the back are forced to work harder to maintain stability, thereby leading to fatigue and strain. Over time, this strain can cause chronic pain and increase the risk of more severe injuries, such as herniated discs.

Orthopaedic pillows help prevent neck injuries by supporting the cervical spine and maintaining its natural curve. A well-designed orthopaedic pillow cradles the neck and head, reducing the likelihood of waking up with a stiff neck or headaches. This support is particularly important for individuals who sleep on their sides, as side sleeping can put additional pressure on the neck and shoulders.

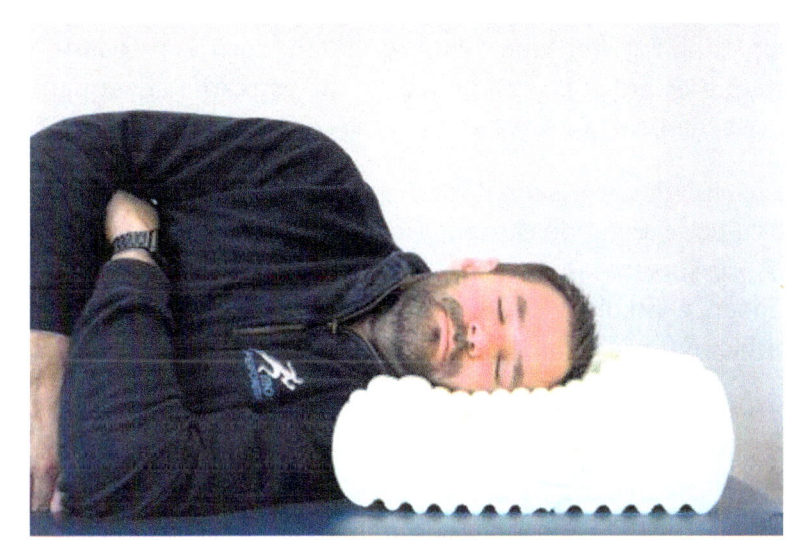

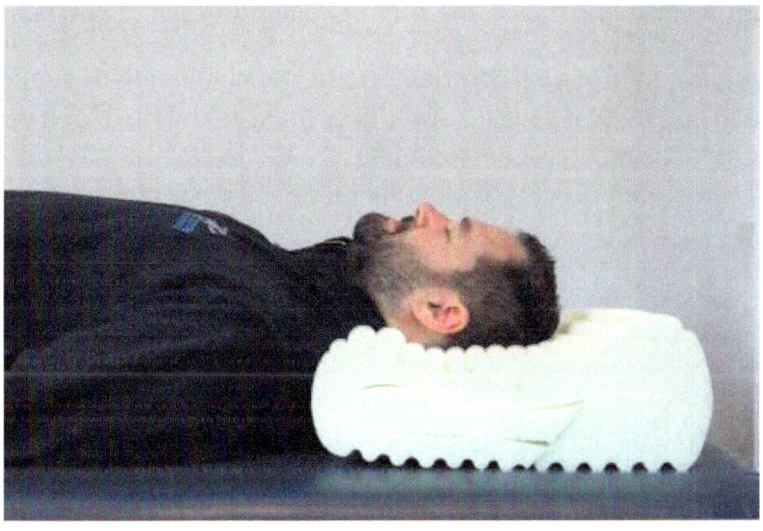

Joint pain is another common issue that can be exacerbated by poor bedding choices. Individuals with arthritis or other joint conditions often find that traditional mattresses and pillows do not provide the support they need, leading to increased pain and discomfort. Orthopaedic bedding can alleviate joint pain by distributing body weight evenly and reducing pressure on the joints.

Orthopaedic mattresses are designed to conform to the body's shape, providing support to the hips, knees, and shoulders. This support helps reduce the pressure on these joints, thereby preventing pain and inflammation. For individuals with conditions such as osteoarthritis or rheumatoid arthritis, an orthopaedic mattress can make a significant difference in quality of sleep and overall comfort.

Proper circulation is essential for overall health and the prevention of injuries. Poor circulation can lead to numbness, tingling, and increased risk of pressure sores. Happily, orthopaedic mattresses and pillows help enhance circulation by reducing pressure points and promoting proper blood flow.

Memory foam and latex mattresses are particularly effective at distributing body weight evenly, reducing the risk of pressure sores and improving circulation. For individuals who are bedridden or have limited mobility, an orthopaedic mattress can be a crucial tool in preventing pressure ulcers and other circulation-related issues.

Orthopaedic pillows also contribute to better circulation by supporting the head and neck in a way that reduces pressure on the blood vessels. This support helps prevent numbness and tingling in the arms and hands, which can occur when the blood flow is restricted during sleep.

Sleep apnoea and other breathing issues can significantly impact quality of sleep and overall health. Orthopaedic pillows are designed to support the head and neck in a way that keeps the airways open, reducing the risk of sleep apnoea and improving breathing.

Elevating the head and neck can help prevent the collapse of the airway, which is a common cause of obstructive sleep apnoea. Orthopaedic pillows with a contoured design help maintain this elevation, promoting better airflow and reducing the likelihood of breathing interruptions during sleep. This support is particularly beneficial for individuals who suffer from snoring or mild to moderate sleep apnoea.

Athletes and active individuals place a higher demand on their bodies and require more restorative sleep to recover from physical exertion. Orthopaedic pillows and mattresses can enhance sleep quality for these individuals by providing the necessary support to prevent injuries and promote recovery.

Proper spinal alignment and pressure relief are crucial for athletes, as they help reduce the risk of injuries and promote muscle recovery. An orthopaedic mattress provides the support needed to alleviate muscle tension and reduce the risk of overuse injuries. Additionally, the improved circulation and pressure distribution offered by orthopaedic bedding can help speed up the recovery process, allowing athletes to perform at their best.

Orthopaedic pillows also benefit athletes by supporting the neck and shoulders, reducing the risk of strain and injury. For individuals who engage in activities that place significant stress on the upper body, such as weightlifting or swimming, an orthopaedic pillow can provide the necessary support to prevent injuries and promote better sleep quality.

Selecting the right orthopaedic pillow and mattress is essential for maximising their benefits. When choosing an orthopaedic mattress, consider factors such as firmness, material, and support. A mattress that is too soft may not provide adequate support, while one that is too firm may create pressure points and discomfort. Memory foam and latex are popular choices for orthopaedic mattresses due to their ability to conform to the body's shape and provide personalised support.

Orthopaedic pillows come in various shapes and sizes, designed to support different sleeping positions. Side sleepers, back sleepers, and stomach sleepers each have specific needs when it comes to pillow support. Side sleepers may benefit from a contoured pillow that supports the neck and keeps the spine aligned, while back sleepers may prefer a pillow that provides support without elevating the head too much. Stomach sleepers, on the other hand, may require a thinner pillow to prevent strain on the neck.

Don't forget, though, that proper maintenance of orthopaedic pillows and mattresses is essential for ensuring their longevity and effectiveness. Regularly cleaning and airing out bedding can prevent the buildup of allergens and extend the life of the materials. Many orthopaedic mattresses come with removable covers that can be washed, making maintenance easier.

Rotating and flipping the mattress periodically can also help maintain its shape and support. This practice ensures that the mattress wears evenly and prevents sagging, which can compromise its orthopaedic benefits. Similarly, orthopaedic pillows should be fluffed and adjusted regularly to maintain their shape and support.

To complicate things further, not all orthopaedic pillows and mattresses be labelled as that. So, it is important that you take your time to select both and that you make sure they are correct for you.

Some up-to-date recommendations for how to choose can be found here:

Focusing on strengthening key areas of the body, enhancing balance, and improving overall fitness, you can become more resilient to the stresses and forces encountered during sport and activity.

Understanding the specific requirements of your sport is essential in this process. Each sport places unique demands on your body and therefore tailoring your injury prevention program to these needs is crucial. This involves adding dedicated injury prevention sessions to your training plan, all of which should complement your usual strength training and sports-specific practice. Screening and re-testing are also vital in identifying weaknesses and tracking improvements over time, ensuring that your prevention program is effective.

However, even with the best preparation, injuries can still occur. This brings us to the next chapter, Injury Treatment, where we'll explore how to manage injuries when they arise and the steps you can take to ensure a safe and efficient recovery.

For access to bonus content and resources, scan this QR Code or visit **https://theweekend-warrior.co.uk/warrior-resources**

Chapter 5: Injury Treatment

Myths and Mistakes

Pain is not an injury or a diagnosis – it is a symptom. Don't make the mistake in thinking that when the pain is gone, so is the injury; you'd be doing yourself a disservice.

Pain is often used as a diagnosis of an injury. Yes, if you have an injury one of the symptoms may be pain, but it is just one of the huge list of signs and symptoms that point towards an actual diagnosis. In fact, there are many times where you can be injured yet feel no pain. There are also times when you have no structural injury, but you are still in pain. I will explain this further, but the important thing to understand is that pain is only part of the problem.

When we talk about injuries it is important that we know a bit more about what pain is: "an unpleasant sensory and emotional experience associated with actual or potential tissue damage, or described in terms of such damage."[5]

Pain is an experience that we feel, so the extent of the damage is not reliably indicated by the amount of pain we experience – everyone is different. We all know people have different "pain thresholds".

Definition of an Injury

"An Injury is damage to a physical part of your body, your feelings, or your reputation"

---

[5] International Association for the Study of Pain. (1979). *Pain terms: A list with definitions and notes on usage*. Pain, 6(3), 249-252

This definition covers a lot of different facets, so for the purpose of this book my definition of an injury is: "anything where a physical structure in the body is damaged or your brain perceives it to be damaged." [6]

There are different types of injuries, some of which are caused by a specific event or mechanism. For example, when someone runs and twists his/her ankle it can be classified as an acute injury. You don't necessarily have to remember the cause for it to be an acute injury; if it was a small injury, or it was a while ago, it can be hard to pinpoint. On the other hand, injuries can be caused by repetitive actions. For example, doing too much road running and causing an overload to your Achilles tendon. There is no specific one-off cause for this kind of injury, rather it is a slow onset of problems that gradually get worse.

Understand the Problem Yourself

To be able to reach your goal, you need to understand what is going on at every stage of your journey. It is important that you understand 'what and why' at each stage of your injury.

For example, you need to know what the diagnosis is and why it is thought to be that. You need to know what the specific treatment is that you'll are getting, what it actually does, and why that is the choice over other things. If you have full understanding at each stage of your injury, it will make it easier to stay on the path. If you just go through the motions, then how do you know it will work? Communication is key to making sure everyone is on the same page and working towards the same target.

---

[6] **Oxford English Dictionary** (2020). *Injury* (2nd ed.). Oxford University Press

Diagnosing an Injury

This is possibly the single most important factor in your journey. If you don't know what the problem is, how can you start to fix it? It would as if your car suddenly stops on the side of the road... you don't know why it has stopped, so you start taking the engine apart but all you needed to do was change the tyre!

Having a clear and correct diagnosis will help you get back to your sport much faster. An unclear or incorrect diagnosis may cause you to focus on the wrong areas and cause the problem to get worse. It will also delay you getting on to the correct path, which may cause other problems.

To get the correct diagnosis it is important that a process is followed and that you or a medical professional do not jump to conclusions. This is precisely what normally leads to an incorrect diagnosis. It is better to take your time in getting the correct diagnosis than rushing this step and following the wrong path before. To get the correct diagnosis, it all starts with getting in front of the right person for the job.

Who to See

I hear a lot of people say that their friend's wife had the same problem as them, so they have just been doing the same sheet of rehab exercise that she was given. Hmmmm... was it an identical injury? Was that friend's injury diagnosed by a professional or simply Dr Google? What was the goal they were trying to reach? And at what stage of their rehab were the targets given? These are amongst a long list of concerns you need to be aware of if you're simply duplicating someone else's rehabilitation schedule.

Don't get me wrong, friends or partners do not want to see people with pain. They have only the best intentions, but it can make injuries significantly worse if they are even slightly wrong. It could also delay the injury being treated properly, thereby making it worse and potentially placing other parts of the body at risk due to overcompensation.

Sometimes you may get lucky, it might work, but it is a complete lottery. Pain translates differently, and every injury is different. Why would the treatment of injuries not be varied in the same way?

And I'm afraid the internet doesn't do much better. Google and social media are the same when it comes to diagnosing an injury. Videos and blogs on the internet are not specific to you. I'm not saying they're all irrelevant, but it is very important that you're directed to the content that is right for you – and that this directive is given by a professional.

There are a lot of professions about, and it can be a nightmare to decide who we need to go and see. Some of the common professions that get thrown around are Dr's/GPs, physiotherapists, osteopaths, sports therapists, chiropractors, massage therapists, surgeons, consultants, etc. The vast number of practitioners out there can make it seem like a minefield. Each profession does have a particular set of skills, so it is important for you to pick the right one for your particular issue. Even though a person comes with a glowing recommendation, it doesn't mean that he/she is the correct person for your problem.

A brain surgeon, though a highly skilled person, wouldn't be the correct person for a hamstring injury. Similarly, a chiropractor wouldn't be the person for a sore throat. They may all get glowing recommendations from the patients they've helped, but will only be the perfect fit for you if they are skilled to fix the problem that you are currently suffering with.

When we are investigating who to see, it's important to know whether they've dealt with any of the problems you're facing yourself. I would suggest that you investigate the type of person the professional normally treats. At Moore Performance Clinics, we are very specialised at helping fitness conscious people and athletes who want to become more active and perform better without pain or the need for painkillers. If you fit into that group, then we are the right fit for you, but if your goals are significantly different then we may be able to help, but it wouldn't be the best fit for you; we would likely send you the right place.

Go to a specialist, not a generalist. Don't forget that, even though you may have tired physiotherapy or another treatment, that doesn't mean that the profession won't help you or that a different physio won't make a difference. Everyone has significantly different areas of specialities within the umbrella of that profession. Any registered profession that has a recognised governing body will require its members to complete a certain number of hours' CPD (continued professional development) training a year – the professional can choose the type. Therefore, someone may have the same degree and title than another, but one person may decide to focus all their time on injuries caused by falls in elderly people, whilst the other may spend their time learning about sports injuries. They will both have the same title but will possess completely different skill sets.

Of course, when deciding who to see you also have to keep cost in mind. As such, the next section focusses on the difference between private and public options.

NHS/ Private

In the UK we are very lucky to have a free healthcare service; the same applies in other countries around the world. In the UK, the National Health Service (NHS) is a brilliant service which provides our population with the facilities to receive medical treatment for anything from a cut all the way through to joint replacements and serious trauma/cancer treatment, all without having to pay a penny. Wonderfully, this includes access to sports injuries and physiotherapy.

In fact, this book's inception came about whilst I was unable to leave the house during the COVID-19 pandemic; the NHS was doing a fantastic job saving lives! We are lucky to have this healthcare system in place here and I will always sing their praises.

It is fair, therefore, that I often get asked why patients should go private when they can get accesses to free health care on the NHS.

I am not going to give you an answer. I am going to help you make the decision based on your goals and the obstacles in your way. For full clarity, my company *Moore Performance Ltd* is a private practice, yet even though it is private I do see people as part of their NHS treatments, and I also refer people to the NHS system on a regular basis... when it is the best thing for their goals.

If money was no object, then our decisions would be a lot easier to make. But for the majority of us, the reality is that money talks. We have to decide if the cost of going private is, firstly, going to give us an outcome relative to our goals, and secondly, whether that outcome would be better if we could see specific people for the specific injury which we are not able to do via the majority of NHS routs? In other words, can the problem be solved significantly quicker and is that worth the money?

Ultimately, going private opens up significantly more options, and therefore, choices. The NHS system takes into account their costs and availability in parallel with what is best for you, which may be the same but not always. Private care gives you complete control over all aspects and allows you to make all the decisions and get as many opinions or options as you would like. The are also a lot more options than most people think available privately, which is not always communicated within the NHS. I would always like to know all of my options when making any decision, especially about my health – so, I would make sure that you know all the options and then you can make the best decision for you, too. If you do not have all the options, you can't be sure you have made the right decision.

These kind of decisions become harder the more they cost. For example, a decision to see a therapist in my clinic will be a lot easier and affordable than deciding on an operation that might cost over £10,000. So, you have to think whether the cost is worth the result. If it means you can play football again, does spending that money give you the result you want? If you do not know the cost, then you have nothing to compare to. Always compare outcomes first... then compare the cost.

Access to the right people is key. As I've mentioned, there are highly skilled people who work for free healthcare systems, but a lot of the time the choice of who we see is very limited and is often decided for you. This may or may not harm your chances of achieving your goal. If your goal doesn't require a high-level procedure, or your injury doesn't require a complex procedure, then it is not as important. But, if you want to compete at a high level or you have a complex injury, then the difference between achieving your goal or not will be down to the surgeon and procedure you choose. So, take your time: decide if the outcome is worth the cost. The NHS doesn't generally let you pick who you see so this is a significant benefit of private care and worth taking into account.

Time is big factor in free healthcare systems; there can often be long waiting lists and significant delays. The reason behind this is because of how things are prioritised. The main way in which this is done is on how serious a problem is and whether it is more serious than another. Depending on the severity, it will get prioritised.

Elective surgeries for sports injuries are therefore not high up on the priority list, as the NHS deals with more serious problems first. This, unfortunately, means that your procedure may take months or years. If you are going privately, however, you will get access to the treatment you need much earlier on. To get an appointment privately, whether that is for a consultation or the procedure itself, is a lot quicker. Some people will still have waiting lists, but often they are nowhere near as long. Consider, therefore, if the cost is worth the speed. If your goal is time sensitive, or if there are check points that you need to hit; this then becomes a significant decision maker.

In summary, deciding whether to go private or not should take you some time. Do enough research and make an informed decision. Always ask yourself whether the outcome is worth the cost.

Scans

One of the most common questions asked by my patients is, "do I Need a scan?"

Before I answer this question, though, I need to gather a lot of information. There is simply so much that people don't understand about scans. Luckily, I'm going to clarify some things.

There are many different types of scans, the most common in sport are the following: X-ray, ultrasound, MRI, and CT. A scan will provide an image of the structures inside the body, and depending on the type of scan, the result will indicate different structures.

X-Ray

This type of imaging can show bone fractures, soft-tissue calcifications, bone spurs, and other issues within the skeletal system. You may go for an **x-ray** if there is a suspected fracture and you want to determine its precise location and severity.

Ultrasound

Ultrasounds use sound waves to create diagnostic images of superficial soft tissues. An ultrasound scan is a way of looking at soft tissues within the body using sound waves rather than radiation. As such. it is thought to be safer than other imaging methods. Scans are used to look at soft tissues in order to determine their size, shape, consistency and any abnormalities. They are particularly useful for tendon injuries, especially tendinopathy (tendonitis) of the Achilles tendon and Patella tendons, as well as muscle injuries. An ultrasound technologist can also conduct imaging in real-time while the body is in motion.

Magnetic Resonance Imaging (MRI)

MRI scans show all tissues within the body, including bones, muscles, cartilage, and fatty tissue. MRI tests are ideal for the diagnostic imaging of muscle injuries, joint damage, ligament sprains and head injuries sustained during sports. This imaging technique uses radio waves within a strong magnetic field to examine the structures of the body.

Computed Tomography (CT)

A CT scanner is a special type of X-ray which uses multiple beams, rather than just the singular one seen in X-rays. The scanner rotates around the patient to give a clearer view of what is happening internally. A CT scan may be ordered if the medical professional requires a more detailed look at the bones or soft tissues. For example, CTs can show fracture lines, loose bodies, and other complications within complex joints. They are also used to look for tumours, bleeding in the brain, aneurysms, lung disease, and internal injuries such as lacerations of the kidneys or spleen.

As you can see from the basic descriptions above, all the scans used in sport do have some similarities. This is why it is important for the patient to be referred by a professional who is experienced in different types of scans. And remember, many of the above scans expose the body to radiation, which in large amounts is detrimental to the body so only in necessary cases should scans be considered.

When you go for a scan, the images are generally taken by a radiographer; these images will then be passed on to a radiologist who will assess and report on what they can see. If you have ever seen a scan, then you will know that they are very different from the colourful diagrams on the wall in medical practices. In reality, the images are very tricky to read without significant experience doing so. What a lot of people don't know is that there is a very large discrepancy between radiologist reports – and this could mean the difference between a clear diagnosis and not.

Some reporting comes down to opinion, which will – of course – differ between different people. Resultantly, a report should not be taken as 100% true, as there may be something missed due to a poor-quality image or simply differing opinions.

Everyone is built slightly differently, and what is normal for one person is not for another. Therefore, when looking at a scan the 'normal' state of the patient must be taken into account. This is in fact very hard to do if only the injured area is scanned. For example, if you scan a knee and find an abnormal joint surface then it will be reported as abnormal. However, the patient may have this exact abnormality on the other side thereby indicating no signs of concern.

As such, a perceived abnormity is not necessarily the cause of a person's pain or problem. Throughout or lives we put a lot of stress on our bodies and we cause damage to structures; it is completely normal to have a degree of damage to parts of the body, much of which does not cause any problem. It is just normal wear-and-tear. Therefore, something that is reported on a scan as abnormal is not necessarily the cause of the problem and should be approached with caution. There is a famous study that demonstrates this point, which I will discuss below.

Table and figure 1 below show a visual representation of a study containing thousands of participants. It is a study into the lower back, specifically looking at problems or abnormalities in peoples' disks, that is, the fluid-filled structures between the bones in our spines. The importance of this study is that none of these participants were suffering or has ever suffered from any back pain. As shown, 52% of people over the age of 30 have disk degeneration with no back pain, and 80% of people over 50 have disk degeneration… also with no back pain. [7]

---

[7] Brinjikji, W., Luetmer, P. H., Comstock, B., Bresnahan, B. W., Chen, L. E., Deyo, R. A., Halabi, S., Turner, J. A., Avins, A. L., James, K., Wald, J. T., Kallmes, D. F., & Jarvik, J. G. (2015). Systematic literature review of imaging features of spinal degeneration in asymptomatic populations. *AJNR. American journal of neuroradiology, 36*(4), 811–816

Table 1: MRI Findings of People WITHOUT Pack Pain

Imaging Finding	Age (years) 20	30	40	50	60	70	80
Disk degeneration	37%	52%	68%	80%	88%	93%	96%
Disk height loss	24%	34%	45%	56%	67%	76%	84%
Disk bulge	30%	40%	50%	60%	69%	77%	84%
Disk protrusion	29%	31%	33%	36%	38%	40%	43%
Facet degeneration	4%	9%	18%	32%	50%	69%	83%
Spondylolisthesis	3%	5%	8%	14%	23%	35%	50%

Figure 1: MRI Findings of People WITHOUT Pack Pain

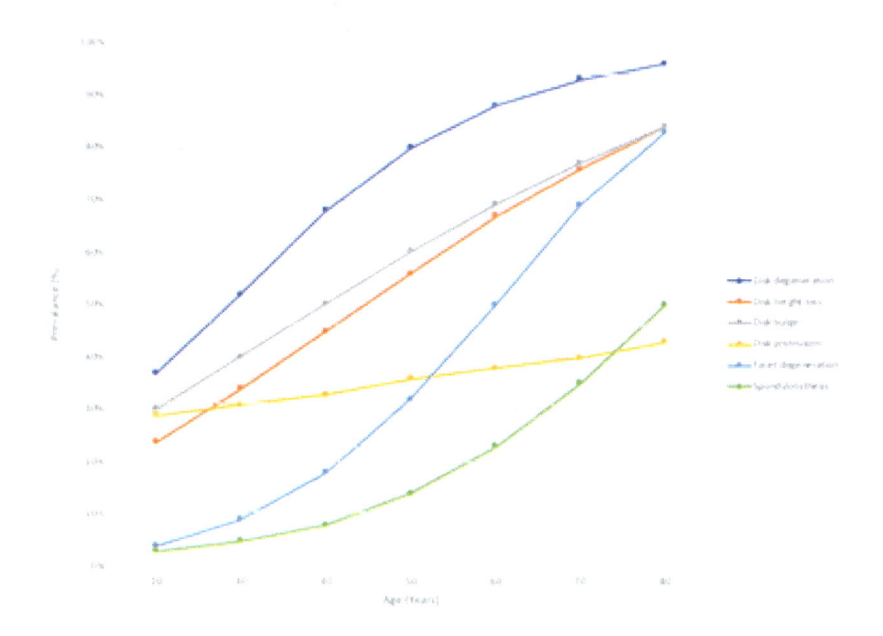

In my clinic I have seen countless people who had an MRI scan and have been told they have something wrong with one of the disks in their spine. Understandably, this is very upsetting for them. Yet, as highlighted by the study above, MRI scans which show issues with these disks are not an indicator of pain. These findings are not signs of "damage", but rather signs of normal aging. So, without symptoms or pain, these MRI findings have very little meaning. Degenerative signs appear to be very common and do not mean that a person will have back pain.

If it is normal to have some degeneration to your lower back structures, please keep in mind that, depending on your age, there is a significant likelihood they scans will report some of these so called 'abnormities'. As these are completely normal to find in people who have no pain, it is unlikely that they are the cause of your problems. Therefore, you don't need to jump into surgery or the like.

Remember, degeneration is completely normal and does not necessarily mean it is the cause of your problem. Therefore, a scan should never be used as a stand-alone diagnostic tool; you risk jumping to a conclusion that might be incorrect.

Don't get me wrong, scanning *is* important and I do refer people for scans regularly, both in my private clinic and in professional rugby teams. But it is important that patients know the above information when getting a scan. For a scan to be used in a meaningful way it should be used as one part of the puzzle, and it should be used in conjunction with a quality subjective assessment where you have a detailed conversation about the mechanism of injury, location and type of pain, and past medical history, etc. This will then be followed by an objective assessment, that is, is a physical assessment of all the structures related the problem. It will involve a number of specific movements and tests.

This will allow the therapist to form a diagnosis which considers everything and is not swayed by a single piece of information from a scan. Scans serve their purpose but must be considered as part of a whole.

Don't Jump to Conclusions!

Treatment Plan

Before a treatment plan has been decided it is crucial that a correct diagnosis is made. A mechanic wouldn't fix the car if he didn't diagnose the problem first, right? That would be like changing the engine when the tyre alone was deflated.

When the problem and contributing factors have been diagnosed it is then time for a treatment plan. And here we come to yet another minefield. Ultimately there is no one-size-fits all treatment, and it's unlikely that a treatment will fix everything – but this all depends on what the problems is.

There are a lot of treatment methods which have become very popular in a short period of time, some of which are good and worthwhile, whilst others are just very good at marketing.

If money is no object, then trying treatments that won't cause harm isn't too much of a problem. Remember, though, that this could exacerbate the problem. And that's why you need to be informed. In my practice, I always use the analogy that, if it isn't used in professional sport, I wouldn't use it in my practice.

I have found the best results occur because of doing the basics right. So, is all of the fancy stuff needed? Sometimes, but not always.

The correct treatment methods should be decided on by a skilled clinician who has a proven track record with regard to your problem and your sport. You wouldn't take your high-performance rally car to a local MOT centre, would you? You would take it to a proven rally mechanic if you wanted to win a stage on the WRC (World Rally Championship).

There are a lot of self-treatment options available to us now. Depending on the current problem you have, and the goal which you are aiming to achieve, you'll have to make a choice. You should always consult your medical professional before trying any self-treatment, no matter what it is. The hard work that is done by a professional in creating a perfect treatment and rehab plan can be undone by using something that you happen to see online or hear about.

Surgery, Injections: The Last Resort

Advancements in medicine has meant we have a lot of options when it comes to treatment, both in terms of non-invasive procedures and invasive ones.

An invasive procedure is "a medical procedure that invades (enters) the body, usually by cutting or puncturing the skin or by inserting instruments into the body".[8] This includes procedures such as operations and injections. These types of procedures carry more risk than those which are non-invasive. Therefore, it is very important that, before you elect to go for an invasive procedure, you have gone through the correct decision-making process.

I am not going to tell you whether to have an invasive procedure or not. Each of us has our own opinion in sports medicine, and that should be decided on a case-by-case basis. As I mentioned earlier, every injury is different; every person's situation and every goal is different. This all needs to be taken into account when deciding which path to go down. Again, if you don't know your destination, how can you plot a path? Make sure your goal is set out otherwise you can't make a logical decision. For example, despite having what seems to be the same injury, no two people will have the same goal – hence they simply will not have the same treatment.

---

[8] **Mosby's Medical Dictionary** (2020). *Invasive procedure*. Elsevier

Ultimately the decision to opt for an invasive surgery is yours, but unless you have enough information to make an informed decision, you can't feel confident. To get this information and make that decision you should start to think about a few things.

Getting in Front of the Correct Person

I've already spoken about this previously, but in the context of this chapter there are some more tactical points that I believe to be key. Not all surgeons and consultants are the same: they use different procedures and have differing material specialities, so picking the right person is vital.

For example, in my practice and in professional rugby there is a list of surgeons that I refer to. They do not all do the same thing, however. When you dig deeper, they are completely different. If 2 people have the same ACL injury (knee ligament injury) – one is a professional rugby player and the other is a recreational cyclist – I would suggest two different consultants who have proven experience in those situations. Obviously, when it comes to a higher impact/twisting sport, the treatment will need to be more robust than a low impact sport, therefore making it more important to have a particular procedure/technique.

There is nothing stopping you from seeing more than one person. Always get a second opinion, because the more you know, the better you'll be able to decide.

Obviously, if you are going private then you will have many more options to pick from. You will need to weigh up if the cost of going private is worth the reward.

And remember, just because you have had a procedure done by a top surgeon doesn't guarantee that you will get back to the level they promised. The procedure is a technical skill that, when done to a high level, gives you the foundations to get to a goal. The rehabilitation after the procedure is crucial!

The main reasons surgeries fail is because of poor or incomplete rehabilitation plans and not because of the actual procedure. Just because a structure has been repaired doesn't mean it is 100%; it needs to heal and strengthen. If you skip stages in your rehabilitation plan you will make the procedure pointless. Read on through the next chapter; it will help you on your path to your goal.

Of course, this decision is ultimately down to you, but you need to have the information from the correct people in order to help you make it. [9]

This chapter laid out some key concepts around understanding pain, diagnosing injuries, and considering treatment options. It's clear that a structured approach, involving the right professionals and taking time to understand your diagnosis, is crucial. You've learned that making assumptions based on pain alone can lead you down the wrong path, and that understanding your treatment options is vital for recovery.

Moving forward, as we delve into the next chapter on **rehabilitation**, we will explore the specific processes that help rebuild strength and function, getting you back to your optimal performance. Rehabilitation is a structured journey, and by the end of it, you'll be well-prepared to return to the sport you love.

Scan the QR code provided for more detailed insights and extra resources. Now, let's move on to building your rehabilitation plan!

---

[9] On a side note, invasive procedures not only have a benefit on the physical structure that is being targeted but there is a big physiological element to having an operation. There have been a couple of studies on placebo surgeries. These studies show have shown a positive result compared to the people who actually had the procedure done. From this, I think it shows how important the mind is in helping to achieve the outcome you desire.

Chapter 6: Rehabilitation

Rehabilitation is "the action of restoring something that has been damaged to its former condition". [10]

The process of rehabilitation should start as early as possible after an injury happens. It should be done in combination with the treatment plan. If an injury is serious enough to require an invasive procedure, then the rehabilitation prior to the operation in order to speed up recovery after the event is equally crucial.

It is vital that there is a plan in place; the plan needs to aim for a goal. Again, if you don't know where you are aiming, it is impossible to build a path to get there.

A rehab plan will often involve a multidisciplinary approach with input from different areas and people. These may include medical professionals (surgeons, physios, etc), strength and conditioners, coaches, etc. Communication is vital when more people are involved in the process. Everyone needs to understand what their role is and what everyone else's role is in the process. If there is complete clarity between everyone, then there is less chance of errors that come from misunderstandings.

Despite the type of injury, the sport, or the level, all injuries follow the same stages of rehabilitation. If any one of them is skipped or not done effectively, it risks significant setbacks or a failed rehab plan.

The Stages of Rehabilitation

There are 5 stages of rehabilitation that I use:

1) Early
2) Intermediate

---

[10] **Mosby's Medical Dictionary** (2020). *Rehabilitation*. Elsevier.

3) Late
4) Return to Training
5) Prevention

Even though these are stages of rehabilitation, these stages are just markers on a continuum that starts with stage 1 – the injury – and finishes when you get back to consistent games or competitions with no lasting signs of that injury. Depending on the injury and the target you have, it will vary as to how long it will take to reach each marker.

There are some overall principles relating to each stage that I will go through; they are general aspects that will be slightly different depending on the injury and the level of the athlete. For some injuries the stages can be worked through quickly, whilst in other cases they could take months to complete.

The Early Stage

This stage starts the moment after your injury occurs. Depending on the severity of the injury and the level in which you are at, this stage in normally under the full control of your medical professional, although there may me some things that other professionals can do. If you do not have a medical professional, then it is a stage which you can manage yourself or with help from someone around you. The goal of the early stage of rehabilitation is to limit damage to the affected structures, avoid other structures becoming involved, pain relief, and to mitigate the inflammatory/chemical responses. These events are important to get under control as soon as possible to avoid complications or delays later down the line. Any delays in this stage will often cause exponential delays moving forward.

POLICE

Protect: The aim is to avoid any further damage to the injured area; this starts with stopping the sport/activity immediately. After you have stopped, the area/joint can be protected with things such as crutches, wheelchairs, and slings which stop any force going through any of the damaged areas. This may also include things such as braces, supports, or boots which will protect the injury. *Protect* in less serious cases does not mean complete immobilisation.

Optimal Loading: This stage requires the correct amount of movement; if done correctly it will help to reduce oedema (swelling) and start to stimulate the healing process in the damaged area. Damaged structures require movement to heal, so if this is done correctly it will drastically improve success at this stage. This can include moving the area yourself (actively), or movement done by a therapist or a device (passively).

ICE: Also known as cryotherapy, this helps to reduce the metabolism of the damaged tissues and therefore stops damage to the cells. Cryotherapy also helps to decrease the sensitivity of the area, thereby decreasing the pain sensations. Applying cryotherapy for extended periods of time can be detrimental to the healing process, however, as it will slow down the cells trying to repair the damage. Damage can also be worsened if blood flow is excessively reduced, and the risk of skin burns and nerve damage increases with prolonged ice application. The prescription for the amount of time to use ice will depend on the injury and severity, but shouldn't be overused. Cryotherapy includes the traditional ice packs – or bag of frozen peas – ice baths, cryocuffs, and cryochambers.

Compression: This is to mitigate the oedema (swelling) and therefore the inflammation process via a reduction to the bleeding in the damaged tissue. The body tends to produce a higher inflammatory response than the injury needs; therefore, reducing this will help to significantly speed up the healing process. We are not trying to stop it – we are controlling it to an optimum level. Compression can be achieved by using a compression bandage: it is importing that it covers the whole of the area and that it is tight enough to compress the, but not too tight that the blood supply is cut off.

Elevation: This will reduce oedema by increasing venous return and therefore facilitating waste removal from the site of injury. This is achieved via suspending the injured limb above the level of the pelvis for the lower body, or above the level of the heart for and upper body.

The POLICE protocol is used for acute injuries, which have a clear moment of injury. If the injury does not have a cause and context (a time/event which you can pinpoint where the injury takes place), but has developed over a period of time, then there is a slightly different way of dealing with it. Compression and elevation would generally not be used.

To move on to the next stage of rehabilitation the pain, oedema, and disfunction should all have improved. If this is not the case then you should not move on to the next phase, as this will risk re-injury.

The Intermediate Stage

This stage comes after the inflammation phase has passed and the body has replaced the damaged structures with similar tissues. At this stage, the resilience and strength of these newly built tissues is low. Thus, the goal of this stage is to restore the range of movement, strength, endurance, balance, and coordination.

Early movement and protective strengthening is crucial to help the alignment of the new structure. It is important that the correct balance is present at this stage; if the plan is too aggressive, it will risk new injuries, setting back the patient. Alternatively, if it is too conservative then the new structures will be disorganised and cause needless adhesions, stiffness, or continued weakness of the area.

Exercises in this stage may start with light force applied to a joint, all without movement; this allows the patient to strengthen structures without risking damage. We can then move on to active movements without any resistance, and ultimately, the patient can move into light resistance exercises either with bodyweight or resistance bands, etc. These exercises start slow and increase in speed as the patient progresses through the stage. Towards the end of this stage the athlete should be fully weightbearing without the need of any brace/support.

Coordination exercises, such as catching, should be incorporated into the training routine at this point. During this time, it's important to continue training the uninjured/healthy parts of the body to prevent overall deconditioning. For example, upper body strength exercises can still be performed if the athlete has a lower leg injury, along with cardio or endurance activities that do not involve the injured area. The focus should be on limiting the athlete regarding their injury, without allowing the rest of their body to lose fitness. This is where a strength and conditioning coach can be creative in designing exercises that avoid the injured area, such as single-leg rowing, for example.

The Late Stage

This is where the tissue has healed but it now needs to be strengthened to cope with the stresses of a particular sport. At this stage, the strengthening is increased to include higher resistances and more complex and functional movements. This will also include jumping and landing movements.

It is in this stage, too, when running is normally added in for lower limb injuries; this is built up throughout the stage. For an upper body injury, this stage will often involve falling exercises. Sport-specific movements are added into this stage; the athlete is normally able to train in their strength or gym sessions as they would normally do, but with a reduced weight/resistance.

The Return to Training Stage

This is when the structures have reached a good level of strength – over 75% that of the opposite side. It is important to note that, at this stage, the athlete is *introduced* to training and not going straight into full training or matches. In a team sport environment, this may start with simply doing the warm-up and then gradually adding controlled drills, then small games, and only then he/she may be ready for full training – though non-contact only. Once all of these are ticked off with no negative consequences, the athlete can then go into full training without restriction. In an individual sport such as running, this stage is a lot simpler, as generally there are fewer external factors; build up the mileage or increase the distances in a controlled fashion.

Remember, just because someone can train doesn't mean they can play or compete. What it does mean is that they are medically fit to train but need to complete a number of full training sessions before competing. It is all too common to see this rushed, the result of which is usually another injury. Build your robustness back up to match/competition fitness.

Generally, the longer you have been out of action, the more your fitness/strengths/speed/balance/skills have decreased, which means you may think you can do what you could before your injury, but the reality is that it may take more time. It is a common occurrence at all levels of sport. People who are injury prone normally skip this step; they are so keen to get back to a competition that they give into pressure and end up hurting themselves again.

Once you have been able to train for the appropriate period of time, you can begin competing again. Remember, though, it may be sensible to limit the first few competitions or games whilst you keep building up your strength and endurance.

From my experience in professional sport and working with athletes, it is not always possible to be able to go through each of these stages as gradually as I would like. Sometimes we are limited by timeframes, competitions, or matches. There will come times where tough decisions need to be made, that is, whether to compete despite not completing the stages – it does come with high risk. Athletes should never take part when it is not safe to do so, but there are some circumstances where one may bend the rules... for example, in a play-off final or a national championship. When this is the case, it is important that everyone knows the risks and assesses whether it is worth it. Being involved may risk a re-occurrence of an injury, a new Injury, reduced performance, or an early finish. So, it is vital that the risks are understood by everyone in order to decide if the outcome is worth the risk; but, it is ultimately the athletes' decision, no one else.

The Prevention Stage

This is begun towards the end of the rehabilitation process, usually when the athlete is integrating into training, and aims at preventing the same injury, or future injuries, from happening. It will involve undertaking a specific injury prevention program that contains exercise/drills to reduce the chance of future injuries. This is the same process as outlined in the injury prevention chapter, but may be extended for more versatility.

Principles of Rehabilitation

Don't Overcomplicate

We all have the tendency of overcomplicating things. When it comes to rehabilitation this often causes more harm than good. All you have to do is scroll through rehab videos on social media to see what I'm talking about; you'll find all sorts of crazy exercises involving multiple pieces of equipment, strange movements, and complicated ques. They may look good on a video, but when you break them down they tend to be just as effective as a very simple movement, one that is easier to master, doesn't need as much equipment, and can be taught easily.

When exercises are simple it is often easier for you to stick to and, as I mentioned in the mindset chapter, we know that consistency will mean that you will experience the snowball effect. Keep things simple, targeted, and easy to execute correctly.

Start Basic and then Progress

Earn the right to progress; if you don't build the foundations then the house will balance on an unstable base. Starting from the beginning is key to being able to progress quickly. Starting simple and basic does not mean that it is going to take longer. It is often quite the opposite. In fact, skipping stages will cause you to go backwards. Why? Because you will have a re-occurrence. It can often be frustrating doing the same exercises over again in particular stages, but it will allow you to keep progressing and avoid setbacks. It is important that you have targets in order to reach the next progression. Again, if you don't know what you're aiming at, how can you work towards it? Having small, short term targets is key for motivation and to make sure that you stay on the correct path. These may include strength, endurance, balance, or range of movement tests that are repeatedly done to see when you have earned the right to move to the next progression.

You Can't Cheat Biology

There is a lot that we can do to provide an injured area with the best environment to heal – protecting, loading, medication, treatment modalities, etc. These all give your body the best chance to heal, but we have to respect that there is only so much we can do to heal structures; sometimes time and patience is needed once you have given the body the best opportunity to heal. If you try and cheat the biology of healing and progress before your body has been able to heal, you will have setbacks. Different structures in the body, such as bone, muscle, ligaments, nerves, etc. all have different ways and speeds in which they heal: don't cheat!

Don't be Afraid to Regress

To reach the goal we need to progress, but if you progress too quickly or recklessly you put yourself at risk of a setback and you might have to start all over again. As I mentioned previously, you should only progress when you hit a certain marker. No one is perfect, though; if you find yourself starting to go backwards, it is crucial that you assess the situation; don't be too hard on yourself.

Be Functional

When we are injured, it is important that we work on our recovery in line with our sport. At any opportunity in the rehab journey, it is very beneficial to relate it back to the skills your sport requires. For example, if you are a netball player ensure that a netball is involved in the rehab session, or a football for a footballer in the same vein. This helps to avoid other skills deteriorating during the injured period.

Use Time to Work on Other Weaknesses/Issues Monitor

If you are injured and are not able to take part in full training or matches, this gives you the time to focus on other things you'd normally not have time to include in your training plan. This is especially true for those longer-term injuries that keep you from your sport for several months. If an injury is serious enough that it is going to keep you out for months, there tends to be a period of immobilisation. So yes, during this time it is important that the main focus remains on protecting the injury and following the rehabilitation schedule for that. But, doing so should not stop you from training other parts of the body.

There is always something you can do when you are injured. If you do not put effort into the parts of your body that are uninjured, then it will mean that the return to your sport is limited by weakness, a general lack of fitness, or fewer skills.

The extent to which you are able to use other parts of the body and systems depends on your exact injury and the restrictions you have to stick to.

To improve performance without doing anything physical involves including things such as performance analysis: videos, playback, conversations, and more. This will provide you with better tactical and technical skills for when you are able to get back into training. It may also include practicing the principles in the mindset and time management chapters.

Rehab Doesn't Stop When You Are Fit to Compete

Rehab should continue despite being back in the game. Just because you are able to compete again it does not mean you are 100%. Even if you are back to the same level that you were pre-injury, that injury happened when you were at 100%, right?

So, you should strive to get to 110% in order to prevent that injury from happening again. As you progress back into competing, much of your rehab should slowly transition into becoming your *prehab*, that is, injury prevention. Prehab exercises should be performed slightly more often than others, at least until you are at that 110% mark. Once you get here and have ticked all the boxes outlined in this chapter, you're well on your way!

In Chapter 6, we've explored the crucial role of **Rehabilitation** in restoring you to full fitness and performance following an injury. Rehabilitation is more than just recovering from an injury, it's about creating a structured plan with clear goals that ensure that you can safely return to your sport without setbacks. The stages of rehabilitation – Early, Intermediate, Late, Return to Training, and Prevention – are a continuous process. Each step builds on the previous one and skipping any part risks re-injury or prolonged recovery.

From the moment an injury occurs, rehabilitation begins. The early stage focuses on protecting the injured area, managing pain, and limiting further damage. As healing progresses, athletes gradually reintroduce movement, build strength, and restore balance and coordination. The later stages involve more functional, sport-specific exercises that prepare the body for the demands of competition.

It's crucial to remember that returning to training does not mean you're immediately ready to compete at full capacity. A gradual, well-monitored transition back to full training ensures athletes can safely regain their pre-injury level of fitness without rushing the process.

With the rehabilitation framework in place, we now move on to the next chapter: Training Methods, where we'll discuss how to enhance athletic performance and prevent future injuries through effective training.

For access to bonus content and resources, scan this QR Code or visit
https://theweekend-warrior.co.uk/warrior-resources

Chapter 7: Training Methods

In the recovery methods chapter, I mentioned that muscles and other structures increase strength/endurance when recovering. Just a recap: during exercise, you cause micro-tears and other forms of damage to structures when you push them hard. After this damage has occurred, your body starts healing. The body does not want structures to be damaged, so when it heals it ultimately becomes slightly stronger. Once you adapt to a given stress, you therefore require additional stress to continue making progress. But, there are limits to how much stress the body can tolerate before it breaks down and risks injury. So, doing too much work too quickly will result in injury or muscle damage, yet doing too little, too slowly will not result in any improvement. There is a delicate balance at play here.

To achieve peak performance in any sport, it is essential to follow a well-structured and effective training program. This chapter explores 10 different methods of training that are specifically designed for semi-professional athletes and high-level amateurs. These methods have been proven to enhance athletic performance, improve physical fitness, and elevate overall skill levels. Additionally, an example training plan will be provided for each method, giving athletes a clear understanding of how to implement these techniques in their own training regime. The regime will depend on the demands of the sport and which type of training you will spend the most time doing, but as I have already outlined in previous chapters, it is important to have a variety of different stresses on the body to make you as robust as possible in your chosen sport.

Sports/Event Specific Training

Sports-specific training is a form of training that focuses on developing the specific skills, physical attributes, and strategies required for a particular sport. It involves tailoring training programs to match the demands and requirements of the sport in order to optimise performance.

By replicating the movements, intensity, and scenarios encountered in the sport, athletes can improve their performance and excel in their chosen discipline. This is often done with a coach or within a team training session, yet individual or small skills can be trained too.

Sports-specific training typically includes the following elements:

1. **Skill Development**: This involves practicing and refining specific skills required for the sport. For example, a football player may focus on dribbling, passing, shooting, and ball control, whilst a tennis player may concentrate on strokes, footwork, and court positioning. Skill development sessions include drills, repetition, and game-specific practice to enhance technique, accuracy, and proficiency.
2. **Physical Conditioning**: Sports-specific training addresses the physical attributes necessary for the sport. This can involve strength training to improve power, speed, and muscular endurance. Conditioning exercises may focus on developing the specific muscle groups and energy systems needed in the sport.

3. **Sport-specific Drills and Simulations**: Training sessions often involve sport-specific drills and simulations to replicate game situations and develop game-specific skills. These drills focus on positioning, timing, communication, and decision-making.

4. **Mental Preparation**: Sports-specific training also includes mental preparation techniques to enhance focus, concentration, and resilience. Athletes may engage in visualisation exercises, goal setting, positive self-talk, and mindfulness techniques to develop mental toughness and handle pressure situations effectively. Refer back to my previous chapter on this.

Sports-specific training is tailored to the individual athlete's needs, position, and goals within the sport. It takes into account the specific physical demands, technical skills, and tactical requirements of the sport. Working with qualified coaches, trainers, and sport-specific experts can help athletes design and implement effective sports-specific training programs.

Speed Training

Speed training is a form of training aimed at improving an athlete's speed and acceleration. It is particularly relevant for sports that require sprinting, rapid changes of direction, or explosive bursts of speed. This obviously is needed in athletics, but is also required in most sports in which you are on your feet – football, rugby, hockey, basketball etc. By incorporating specific exercises and drills, speed training can enhance an athlete's ability to generate power, react quickly, and maintain high-speed movements.

The primary goal of speed training is to improve an athlete's running mechanics, including things such as contact time, stride length and stride frequency. This involves developing strength and power in the lower body, optimising body positioning and posture, and refining the coordination and timing of movement patterns.

One of the key aspects of speed training is developing explosive power. Strength exercises such as plyometrics, which involve rapid and powerful muscle contractions, are commonly used to enhance the stretch-shortening cycle of the muscles. The stretch-shortening cycle is a process where muscles quickly stretch and then contract, using stored energy to enhance power and efficiency in movements like a spring coils. These exercises can include squat jumps, box jumps, bounding, or depth jumps. By training the muscles to generate force quickly, athletes can improve their ability to accelerate rapidly and reach top speeds.

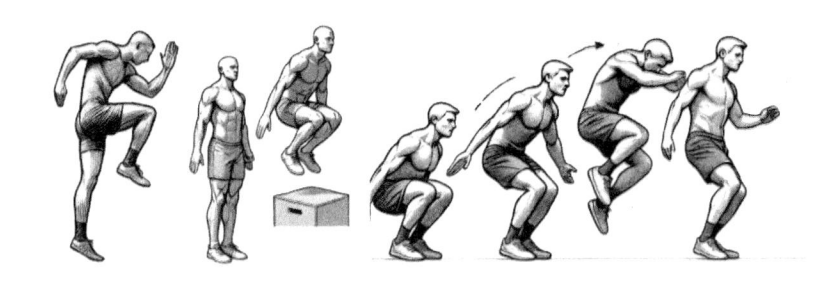

Another important component of speed training is technique work. This includes focusing on proper running form, arm swing, foot strike, and body position. Coaches and trainers often provide feedback and guidance to athletes to optimise mechanics and minimise any wasted movements or energy. Drills like high knees, butt kicks, or A-skips can be incorporated to reinforce proper running mechanics and improve stride efficiency.

Speed training is highly sport-specific, with different sports emphasising various aspects of speed. For example, sprinters require explosive acceleration and top-end speed, whilst team sports like football or tennis may focus on short bursts of acceleration. Therefore, speed training should be tailored to the specific demands of the sport and the individual athlete's needs.

In addition to drills and exercises, speed training often includes interval training. This involves alternating periods of high-intensity sprints with periods of active recovery or rest. Interval training not only improves an athlete's speed but also enhances cardiovascular fitness and muscular endurance.

Examples of speed training drills include:

1. Acceleration sprints: Athletes start from a stationary position and progressively increase their speed over short distances, focusing on quick and powerful acceleration.
2. Ladder drills: Using an agility ladder on the ground, athletes perform rapid footwork patterns, such as high knees, lateral hops, or quick steps. This helps improve foot speed and coordination.

3. Shuttle runs: Athletes sprint back and forth between two markers, emphasising rapid changes of direction, acceleration, and deceleration.
4. Hill sprints: Running uphill forces athletes to exert more power and effort, improving leg strength and power output.

It is essential to note that speed training should be implemented gradually and with proper warm-ups, adequate stretching, and a focus on maintaining proper technique throughout the training sessions.

Cardiovascular Endurance

Cardiovascular training, also known as aerobic or cardio training, focuses on improving the body's ability to efficiently transport oxygen to the muscles and sustain prolonged physical activity. It primarily targets the cardiovascular system, including the heart, lungs, and circulatory system. Cardiovascular training plays a crucial role in enhancing endurance, stamina, and overall aerobic fitness.

The main goal of cardiovascular training is to elevate the heart rate and sustain it at a moderate to high intensity for an extended period. This continuous and repetitive movement works the heart and lungs, increasing their efficiency and capacity. Over time, the cardiovascular system adapts by becoming more efficient at delivering oxygen and nutrients to the working muscles while removing waste products.

Cardiovascular training is relevant for a wide range of sports and activities that require endurance, such as distance running, cycling, swimming, rowing, and team sports like football or rugby. It is also beneficial for overall health and fitness, as it helps reduce the risk of cardiovascular diseases, improves lung function, and aids in weight management.

There are various forms of cardiovascular training, each with its own benefits and considerations:

1. Continuous training: This involves maintaining a steady pace of moderate intensity exercise for an extended duration. Activities like jogging, cycling, or swimming at a steady pace for 30 minutes or longer form part of this. It improves aerobic endurance and is a good starting point for beginners.
2. Interval training: Interval training alternates between periods of high-intensity effort and recovery or lower-intensity activity: sprinting for a set distance or time, followed by a period of walking or slow jogging, for example. Interval training challenges both aerobic and anaerobic systems, improving cardiovascular capacity and increasing speed. It is particularly relevant for sports that involve intermittent bursts of high-intensity effort, such as football, tennis, or basketball.
3. Fartlek training: Fartlek, meaning "speed play" in Swedish, involves incorporating bursts of speed or intensity into continuous training. It involves varying the pace and intensity throughout the workout, such as increasing speed during specific intervals or incorporating sprints into a longer run. Fartlek training helps develop both aerobic and anaerobic fitness, enhancing speed, endurance, and the ability to handle changes in pace during sports.
4. Cross-training: Cross-training involves engaging in different types of cardiovascular exercises to vary the stress on the body and prevent overuse injuries. It can include activities like swimming, cycling, rowing, or using elliptical machines. Cross-training helps improve overall cardiovascular fitness, reduces the risk of repetitive strain injuries, and provides variety in training routines.

It is important to gradually increase the duration and intensity of cardiovascular training to avoid overexertion and minimise the risk of injury. Athletes should listen to their bodies, allow for adequate rest and recovery, and consider consulting with a fitness professional or coach to develop a well-rounded cardiovascular training program.

Athletes who compete in sports that do not necessarily require cardiovascular endurance, for example golf or snooker, will often include cardiovascular exercise within their plan; it has been proven to be helpful in improving mental health, managing weight, and improving all-round physical health. This then allows them to focus and improve on the elements they require for their sport.

Change of Direction and Agility

Change of direction and agility training are crucial components of many sports; both focus on an athlete's ability to quickly and efficiently change direction, accelerate, decelerate, and manoeuvre through various movements and obstacles. These training methods enhance an athlete's agility, speed, coordination, and overall movement capabilities. They are particularly relevant for sports that involve rapid changes in direction, quick steps, and agility-based movements.

The primary goals are to improve an athlete's ability to change direction quickly, maintain balance and body control during dynamic movements, and execute precise movements with speed and accuracy. These skills are essential for athletes to evade opponents, react to game situations, and perform sport-specific movements effectively.

There are various approaches and exercises used in change of direction and agility training, including:
1. Cone drills: Setting up a series of cones or markers in different patterns, athletes perform various movements such as shuttle runs, figure-eight runs, T-drills, or box drills. These drills improve agility, change of direction, and body control.
2. Ladder drills: Using an agility ladder on the ground, athletes perform quick footwork patterns, such as lateral movements, high knees, or lateral hops. These drills improve foot speed, coordination, and agility.
3. Reactive agility drills: These drills involve reacting to external cues or signals, such as visual or auditory cues, and quickly changing direction or performing specific movements. This

improves reaction time, decision-making, and agility under dynamic conditions.
4. Mirror drills: Athletes work in pairs, mirroring each other's movements. One athlete leads with a series of movements, and the other follows and mimics those movements in real-time. This drill enhances agility, coordination, and the ability to anticipate and react to movements.
5. Sport-specific agility drills: These drills replicate movements and scenarios encountered in the specific sport. For example, soccer players may practice quick changes of direction while dribbling or reacting to visual cues, while basketball players may focus on lateral movement and defensive slide drills.

It is important to incorporate a variety of change of direction and agility exercises into training routines to promote comprehensive development. Athletes should focus on proper form, technique, and body control while performing these exercises to maximise their effectiveness and reduce the risk of injury.

Consistency, progression, and specificity are key in change of direction and agility training. Athletes should gradually increase the complexity and intensity of the exercises as their skills improve. This will continuously challenge their agility, change of direction, and reactive abilities, thereby enabling them to perform at a higher level in their respective sports.

Gym/Strength Training

Strength training, also known as gym or weight training, plays a vital role in enhancing athletic performance and overall physical fitness. It involves exercises and techniques aimed at increasing muscular strength, power, and endurance through the use of resistance such as weights, machines, or bodyweight.

The main objective of strength training is to stimulate muscle adaptation, which is the growth and strengthening of muscle fibres. As mentioned earlier, by subjecting the muscles to progressively heavier loads, strength training induces micro-tears in the muscle fibres. During the recovery process, the body rebuilds these fibres to be stronger and more resistant to future stress, leading to increased strength and muscle mass.

Strength training is relevant and beneficial for athletes across various sports. It helps improve performance in activities that require explosive power, such as sprinting, jumping, and throwing. Additionally, strength training can enhance endurance by increasing muscular stamina and delaying the onset of fatigue. It is also effective in injury prevention and rehabilitation, as stronger muscles provide better support and stability to the joints and surrounding structures.

When designing a strength training program, it is crucial to consider the specific demands of the sport and the individual athlete's needs and goals. The exercises and techniques selected should align with the movements and muscle groups utilised in the sport. Additionally, the program should be progressively challenging, gradually increasing the intensity, volume, and complexity of the exercises over time.

Examples of strength training exercises include compound movements such as squats, deadlifts, bench presses, and pull-ups, which engage multiple muscle groups simultaneously. Isolation exercises, such as bicep curls or calf raises, target specific muscles or muscle groups. The program may also incorporate plyometric exercises, which involve explosive movements like box jumps or medicine ball throws to develop power and agility.

To ensure safety and maximise benefits, good form and technique are essential during strength training. Athletes should learn and practice correct lifting mechanics, including proper body alignment, breathing techniques, and control of the weights. Working with a qualified strength and conditioning coach can help athletes develop proper technique, prevent injuries, and optimise their training outcomes.

Coordination/Reaction

Coordination and reaction training are essential components of development, focusing on enhancing an athlete's ability to move efficiently, react quickly, and coordinate their movements effectively. These training methods improve agility, balance, spatial awareness, and overall motor skills. They are particularly relevant for sports that require precise movements, rapid decision-making, and quick reflexes.

The main goals of coordination and reaction training are to improve neuromuscular communication, enhance proprioception (awareness of body position and movement), and develop the ability to respond quickly and accurately to stimuli. These skills are crucial for athletes to perform complex movements, maintain balance, and react swiftly to changes in the environment or opponents' actions.

Coordination and reaction training are required across a wide range of sports, including team sports such as soccer, basketball, or hockey, and individual sports like tennis, martial arts, or gymnastics. They are also beneficial for everyday activities that require coordination and quick reactions.

There are various approaches and exercises used in coordination and reaction training, including:

1. Agility ladder drills: Using an agility ladder on the ground, athletes perform various footwork patterns, such as quick steps, lateral movements, or high knees. These drills improve foot speed, coordination, and agility.
2. Cone drills: Setting up a series of cones or markers, athletes perform rapid changes of direction, weaving in and out, or performing figure-eight patterns. Cone drills enhance agility, body control, and spatial awareness.
3. Reaction ball exercises: Using a small, unpredictable bouncing ball, athletes react quickly to catch or strike the ball in different directions. This improves hand-eye coordination, reaction time, and reflexes.

4. Mirror drills: Athletes work in pairs, mirroring each other's movements. One athlete leads with a series of movements, and the other follows and mimics those movements in real-time. This drill enhances coordination, body awareness, and synchronicity with a partner.
5. Sport-specific drills: These drills mimic movements and scenarios encountered in a specific sport. For example, tennis players may practice rapid lateral movements and quick changes of direction, while basketball players may focus on defensive slide drills or reaction to passes.
6. Balance and stability exercises: These exercises involve activities that challenge balance and stability, such as single-leg balances, balance board exercises, or stability ball exercises. Improving balance and stability contributes to overall coordination and movement control.

It is important to incorporate a variety of coordination and reaction exercises into training routines to promote comprehensive development. Athletes should focus on form and technique while performing these exercises to maximise their effectiveness and reduce the risk of injury. Athletes should gradually increase the difficulty and complexity of the exercises as their skills improve. This will continuously challenge the neuromuscular system and further enhance coordination, reaction time, and agility.

Flexibility/Mobility

Flexibility and mobility training focuses on improving joint range of motion, muscle elasticity, and recovery. These training methods are essential for athletes as they enhance performance, reduce the risk of injuries, and improve overall movement quality. Flexibility refers to the ability of a muscle or group of muscles to lengthen, while mobility refers to the joint's ability to move freely and through its full range of motion.

The primary goals of flexibility and mobility training include increasing joint flexibility, improving muscle elasticity, and correcting muscle imbalances. By incorporating this into the plan, athletes can optimise their movement efficiency, prevent muscle imbalances, and maintain proper posture and alignment.

Flexibility and mobility training are relevant for athletes across various sports, as well as for general fitness and well-being. Sports that involve extensive ranges of motion, such as gymnastics, martial arts, dance, or yoga, benefit from these training methods. However, athletes in all sports can enhance their performance and reduce the risk of injuries by improving their flexibility and mobility.

There are different approaches and techniques for flexibility and mobility training, including:

1. Static stretching: This involves holding a stretch position for a certain duration, typically around 30 seconds or longer. Static stretching helps improve muscle length and joint flexibility. It is commonly performed after a workout or during a separate stretching session.
2. Dynamic stretching: Dynamic stretching involves moving through a full range of motion in a controlled manner. It activates the muscles and prepares them for movement. Dynamic stretches can mimic movements used in the sport or activity, such as leg swings, arm circles, or walking lunges.
3. Proprioceptive Neuromuscular Facilitation (PNF): PNF stretching techniques involve a combination of static stretching and isometric contractions. It is performed with a partner or using resistance to achieve greater gains in flexibility. PNF stretching techniques include contract-relax stretching and hold-relax stretching – a qualified person is often required when doing this.
4. Foam rolling: Foam rolling, also known as self-myofascial release, is a self-massage technique using a foam roller. By applying pressure to specific areas, athletes can release tension, improve muscle elasticity, and increase joint range of motion.

5. Yoga and Pilates: Yoga and Pilates incorporate a variety of movements and poses that enhance flexibility, mobility, and body awareness. These practices focus on strength, balance, and flexibility while promoting mind-body connection.

When implementing flexibility and mobility training, athletes should consider their individual needs and goals. It is important to start gradually, focusing on proper form and technique to prevent injury. Regular and consistent training is key to improving flexibility and mobility over time.

This is a type of training that, interestingly, those in team sports don't like to do, but it is crucial to be able to use your body and move in the most efficient way for your sport. Missing this form of training is often why athletes will not progress in other types of training or will get injured.

Cross-Training

As mentioned in a previous chapter, cross-training is a training approach that involves a variety of different exercises, activities, or sports to complement an athlete's primary training regimen. It aims to provide a well-rounded fitness foundation, prevent overuse injuries, and enhance overall performance. Cross-training includes activities that are different from the athlete's primary sport in terms of movement patterns, intensity, and impact.

The main goals of cross-training are to improve overall fitness, prevent burnout, reduce the risk of overuse injuries, and provide mental and physical variety. Cross-training provides a mental break from the routine of the primary sport, helping athletes avoid burnout and maintain enthusiasm for training. Exploring new activities can be enjoyable and provide a fresh perspective on fitness. Incorporating diverse activities, athletes can target different muscle groups, improve cardiovascular fitness, and maintain motivation throughout their training journey.

It's important to tailor cross-training activities to complement an athlete's primary sport and goals. Athletes should consider their individual needs, fitness levels, and the potential impact of cross-training activities on their primary sports.

Cross-training typically includes the following elements:

1. Diversity of activities: Cross-training involves engaging in activities that are different from the athlete's primary sport. For example, a runner might cross-train by cycling, swimming, or doing yoga. This provides a break from repetitive motions and allows muscles and joints used in the primary sport to recover while still maintaining fitness.
2. Low impact options: Cross-training often includes low-impact activities to give joints a break from the repetitive strain experienced in some sports. Swimming, cycling, and using elliptical machines are examples of low-impact exercises that maintain cardiovascular fitness without putting excessive strain on joints.
3. Active recovery: Cross-training can also serve as a form of active recovery on rest days. Engaging in light activities such as walking, gentle stretching, or easy swimming helps promote blood circulation, reduce muscle soreness, and aid in recovery.
4. Skill transfer: Some activities in cross-training can have skills that transfer to the primary sport. For example, participating in table tennis will help hand-eye coordination for sports such as rugby.

Tactical/Analysis

Tactics and analysis are essential components of overall athletic development. It involves reviewing past performances, learning about the sport, studying the opposition, and analysing the strategies and techniques employed by top athletes and teams. This type of training is primarily conducted in a classroom environment, where athletes can delve into the intricacies of their sport and gain a deeper understanding of its nuances.

The purpose of tactical training is multifaceted. Firstly, it allows athletes to evaluate their own performances and identify areas for improvement. By studying video footage or analysing statistical data, athletes can pinpoint weaknesses in their game or identify patterns of play that could be exploited. Additionally, this helps athletes gain a comprehensive understanding of their sport. By learning about the history, rules, and strategies of the game, athletes can develop a broader perspective and make more informed decisions. This knowledge also allows athletes to anticipate their opponent's moves and adapt their own strategies accordingly.

Studying the opposition is a crucial aspect of tactical training, by analysing the strengths and weaknesses of rival teams or athletes, athletes can formulate game plans and tactics to gain a competitive edge. This type of training helps athletes identify patterns of play, study individual players' tendencies, and devise strategies to exploit weaknesses or neutralise strengths.

Tactical training is relevant across a wide range of sports, particularly those that involve strategic decision-making, team coordination, and quick thinking. Team sports such as football, rugby, and hockey heavily rely on tactical analysis to devise effective game plans and make in-game adjustments. Individual sports like tennis, golf, and boxing also benefit from this, as athletes need to stay focused, adapt to changing conditions, and outthink their opponents.

Examples of tactical sessions may include watching footage and analysing player movements, studying the tactics employed by successful teams or athletes, engaging in discussions and brainstorming sessions to develop new strategies, and engaging in visualisation exercises to improve mental focus and concentration. This is often done by using different technologies.

Most tactical analysis has been done through simply recording videos and then watching them back slowly; one can also draw lines/diagrams over this content. It can can also include attaching sensors to equipment or the athlete himself/herself to capture data such as movement patterns, speed, etc. No matter what you choose, I would always recommend starting with the basics and by reviewing video recordings, even if this is on your own phone. Don't spend vast amounts of money straight off the bat. Technology changes very quickly – invest only when you're sure.

Mental/Psychological Training

Mental training is another critical type of training. It involves techniques and exercises aimed at enhancing an athlete's mental resilience, focus, and concentration. Mental training can include visualisation exercises, mindfulness techniques, goal-setting strategies, and psychological skills training. By developing a strong mental game, athletes can improve their performance under pressure, maintain composure in challenging situations, and enhance their overall competitive mindset, as mentioned in earlier chapters.

As with the tactical training above, mental training does not require burning physical energy and is therefore to forget about. But, never forget that this is arguably the most important type of training and may well have the biggest impact on your performance.

As this does not require lots of equipment and facilities, most mental/physiological training then can also be the easiest to fit into your plan. This type of training requires an open mind and a willingness to change the way in which you may have been told to think. There is not a single professional athlete who doesn't spend a significant amount of time improving their mental capability, and I would be confident in saying that the people who spend the most time training their brain are the people who have the most success.

Training Methods is an essential aspect of improving performance. Training is about a delicate balance, while pushing your body to adapt to new stresses, you must also avoid overtraining, which can lead to injury. Conversely, doing too little will result in stagnation. This chapter outlines key methods for enhancing strength, endurance, agility, and sport-specific skills, focusing on everything from speed training to cardiovascular endurance, gym workouts, coordination drills, and much more.

In my clinics, I emphasise the importance of **sport-specific training**, where you tailor workouts to meet the unique demands of their chosen sport. This can include practicing precise skills, enhancing physical conditioning, and refining techniques that simulate real-game scenarios. We also cover the importance of strength training, flexibility, mobility, and cross-training, all of which are crucial to building a robust and versatile athlete capable of handling various physical challenges.

As you continue to improve and push your limits, keep in mind that training methods must evolve. It's not just about repetition, but variety, incorporating mental and tactical training alongside physical work can be the key to staying ahead in competition.

Up next is "Recovery Strategies", where you'll learn how to maximise rest and recovery to ensure you stay injury-free and improve faster!

For a deeper dive into these techniques and examples of training plans, simply scan the QR code.

Chapter 8: Recovery Strategies

In sport, especially when working and juggling a busy life, recovery is normally the first thing that gets skipped. It is often not the most interesting aspect of training and, yes, we don't love our chosen sport because the recovery sessions are enjoyable. But, getting the recovery right allows you to be at your best when you train or compete; it's entirely necessary.

Recovery is critical to sports performance for many different reasons. This is truth when it comes to both physiological and psychological factors. Rest is necessary so that the muscles can repair, rebuild and therefore strengthen, but it is also necessary for your mind to rest.

Exercise or any physical work puts stress on the body and causes depletion of energy stores, muscle breakdown, and the loss of fluid. Building recovery into a training program is important; this is the time that structures adapt to the stress of exercise and the effects of training take place. Recovery allows the body to replenish energy stores and repair damaged tissues. In fact, recovery allows these stores to be replenished and allows tissue repair to occur. Without sufficient time to repair, the body will just continue to breakdown and therefore you won't improve.

In an earlier chapter, I mentioned how our muscles and other structures increase their strength/endurance etc. Just to recap: during exercise you cause microtrauma and other forms of damage to structures when pushing them hard. After this damage has occurred, your body catches on and is then set on healing. The body does not want structures to be damaged, so when it heals these structures, it heals them slightly stronger. This is called adaptation to exercise. Once you adapt to a given stress, you require additional stress to continue to make progress. If you don't allow structures to adapt, then they will not be able to cope with the same level of stress and will therefore breakdown, thereby significantly increasing the risk of injury.

There are two categories of recovery. First is immediate/short-term recovery, that is, recovery from a particularly intense training sessions or an event/match. The second is long-term recovery and it needs to be built into your whole season or year's training schedule. Both are very important for performance.

Short-term recovery happens in the hours and days immediately after intense exercise, which may include a training session or a match/tournament/event. This generally starts with some form of active recovery and involves low-intensity exercise after workouts. Another major focus of short-term recovery is replenishing energy stores and lost fluids. During this time the soft tissues start removing chemicals that build up as a by-product of energy usage during exercise. Of course, adequate, quality sleep is another crucial part of this short-term phase of your recovery.

Long-term recovery refers to the strategies that are built into the long-term season/yearly training program. Training schedules will include recovery days and weeks during which you will have a significant reduction in intensity. You cannot cope with high levels of physical or mental stress all day, everyday, without breaking down. Rest is vital.

Do the Simple Things Well

Before I delve into some of the current tried and tested methods of recovery, I want to go back to something I mentioned many times so far: **do the simple things well**. Recovery is an area of new research and new products, and it will always be so. It is therefore important that, whatever method you choose, has been tried and tested. But even so, if you don't do the simple free, recovery methods correctly then costly machines are not going to get you anywhere near your potential.

It is also important to know that recovery plans will not always be perfect. We all get into sport because we enjoy it, and a big part of that is the social aspect of being a part of a team/club/venue etc. For example, if you are part of a rugby team there is nothing wrong with having a few beers after the game, but you need to realise it is not going to help your recovery. Therefore, plan it accordingly. If you have just had a semi-final and the final is the following week, then it would not be sensible to do drink 10 pints, right? Be sensible.

I am now going to delve into some of the specific recovery strategies that have been used in sport for a long time.

Planning

To make sure you peak at the right time you need to schedule it. Yes, that's right. When you know the time you need to be at the top of your game, you can schedule in more recovery leading up to your goal. When you plan your recovery sessions, you need make sure they are blocked out in your diary in the same way that a regular team-training or gym session might be. Re-read the time management section of this book to make sure you're on board.

Engaging

Recovery is often the session that is classed as boring. These sessions generally lack a competitive nature and they don't push the body to its maximum, an aspect of training that athletes often aspire to. So, change the game! The easiest thing to add to recovery sessions is some form of cross-training as part of the recovery process. For example, the England football famously swimming with inflatable unicorns during the 2018 World Cup; this created great engagement from the players – it also allowed them to get the benefits of hydrotherapy. Rugby teams in Australia are famous for doing their recovery on the beach for the same reasons. From my experience, the more you are engaged and enjoying it, the better the recovery session will be. Creativity is key.

Stretching and Mobility

Beyond improving flexibility and range of motion, these practices play a significant role in aiding the body's recovery process. One of the primary benefits of stretching and mobility exercises as a recovery method is their ability to alleviate muscle tension and soreness. As previously mentioned, intense activity can lead to the accumulation of muscle tightness and micro-tears. Engaging in targeted stretches helps to release this tension, allowing muscles to relax and recover more efficiently. By increasing blood flow to the muscles, stretching promotes the delivery of vital nutrients and oxygen which are essential for repair and recovery.

Stretching and mobility exercises also assist in improving circulation and lymphatic drainage. Lymphatic fluids carry waste products away from muscle tissues. Gentle stretching aids in stimulating the lymphatic system, thereby enhancing the removal of metabolic waste and reducing inflammation. This reduction in inflammation is key to promoting a faster recovery and minimising the discomfort associated with post-exercise muscle soreness.

Enhancing flexibility through stretching also contributes to injury prevention. Inflexible muscles are more prone to strains and other injuries. Regular stretching and mobility work helps maintain an optimal range of motion, ensuring that muscles and joints can move freely without unnecessary strain. This increased flexibility promotes better biomechanics and reduces the risk of overuse injuries that could hinder an athlete's performance and progress.

Incorporating mobility exercises into a recovery routine also improves joint health. As athletes engage in high-impact sports, joints undergo significant stress. Mobility exercises help maintain joint integrity by lubricating the joint capsule, thereby enhancing synovial fluid circulation and promoting better shock absorption. Well-mobilised joints are less likely to experience stiffness and discomfort, allowing athletes to move more effectively in their chosen sport.

Beyond the physical benefits, stretching and mobility exercises also contribute to mental recovery. Post-sport activities often leave athletes feeling fatigued and mentally drained. Engaging in a focused stretching routine provides a mental break, allowing athletes to unwind, decompress, and promote a sense of relaxation. The meditative aspects of stretching help reduce stress levels and promote a positive mindset, which are crucial for long-term athletic success.

To effectively incorporate stretching and mobility exercises into a recovery routine, you should consider the following:

- Consistency: Regularity is key. Including stretches and mobility exercises in both pre- and post- sport routines ensures that muscles and joints are well-prepared for activity and that they recover optimally afterwards.
- Tailored Approach: Focus on stretches that target muscle groups and joints commonly used in your sport. A customised approach ensures that recovery efforts are aligned with the specific demands of your activity.
- Gradual Progression: Avoid aggressive stretches that could lead to injury. Gradually increase the intensity of stretches to prevent overstretching and strains.
- Quality over Quantity: Focus on proper form and technique during stretches. A controlled, mindful approach maximises the benefits and minimises the risk of injury.
- Group or partnered: Doing this with a group, or at least on other person, will provide a distraction and keep you accountable.

Hydrotherapy

Hydrotherapy is the use of a swimming pool for exercises. A swimming pool can be a valuable training and recovery tool when used the right way. Pool recovery sessions have been popular with elite athletes for a long time – so if it works for them, why not you? Part of what makes pool recovery workouts so effective is that they let you put your body through a controlled range of motion without any of the impacts inherent in dry land training.

The swimming pool's hydrostatic pressure plays a crucial role in recovery. Hydrostatic pressure is the force exerted by water on all immersed objects. When athletes submerge themselves in the pool, hydrostatic pressure aids in reducing swelling and oedema by assisting the body's natural mechanisms of fluid movement. This pressure also promotes better blood circulation, leading to improved oxygen and nutrient delivery to muscle tissues and ultimately speeding up the recovery process.

Furthermore, the cooling effect of the water draws heat away from muscles, reducing inflammation and promoting vasoconstriction. This is particularly effective for alleviating muscle soreness after intense workouts. By alternating between periods of floating in the water and performing gentle movements, athletes can encourage the circulation of oxygen-rich blood to muscle tissues, aiding in the removal of metabolic waste products and promoting recovery.

Active recovery in water fosters improved joint range of motion. The buoyancy of water allows athletes to move through a wider range of motion than they might be able to achieve on land. This gentle stretching and movement encourage flexibility and maintain joint mobility, which are vital components of an effective recovery process.

In terms of hydrotherapy, a program of about 20-30 minutes is ideal for the recovery process. *THE FOLLOWING ROUTINE IS DESIGNED FOR A SHORT SWIMMING POOL WITH A LENGTH OF ABOUT 20 METRES AND A DEPTH THAT IS BELOW CHEST LEVEL.*

Using the side of the pool for support if needed, begin by performing:

- Forward **Leg Swings** — 2x10 each leg
- Sideways **Leg Swings** — 2x10 each leg

After the Leg Swings, move to the *movement* portion of the routine. This simple routine consists of nine laps using various movements:

- Forward Jog down, Backpedal back
- Forward Jog down, Backpedal back
- High Knees down, Carioca back
- Butt Kicks down, Forward Skips back
- High Knees down, Carioca back (facing other direction)
- Freestyle swim down, Shuffle back
- Freestyle swim down, Shuffle back (facing opposite way)
- Breast stroke down, Lateral Skip back
- Breast stroke down, Lateral Skip back

It's that simple. This short routine can stimulate recovery and leave you feeling better than you did before.

Scan this code to see me walking you through this session on the free resources page.

Playing a game such as pool basketball, pool volleyball, tag, or water polo allows you to have fun and blow off steam whilst stimulating recovery. Games put you through a wide variety of movements and motions, which accelerate recovery and help flush out lactic acid whilst keeping impact to a minimum.

Sleep

Sleep is a key aspect to recovery. Previously, I mentioned the autonomic nervous system; think back to when I mentioned the 'rest and digest' state, that is, the time when the body heals and repairs damage. As the name suggests, in this state we are able to digest food efficiently. During this state, sleep comes into its own. Sleep is essential for everyone, but it is even more important for athletes to meet the physical and mental demands of their sport. All the way from the recreational level to the elite, anyone looking to perform at the top of their game needs to make sleep a priority.

Most people need about 6-8 hours of sleep a night. If you're an athlete in training, you need more. In the same way that athletes need more calories when they're in training, you also need more sleep.

As an athlete, you put more stress on your body than most, and therefore you need more time to recover and repair. It is recommended that athletes sleep for 8-10 hours. It is documented that world class athletes Roger Federer and LeBron James sleep for an average of 12 hours a night, whilst Usain Bolt, Venus Williams, and Maria Sharapova get up to 10 hours a night. But remember, it is not just the *quantity* of sleep that is important – the *quality* is also key.

A study tested basketball players after 5-7 weeks of increasing their sleep to 10 hours per night. The results? Shooting accuracy improved by 9% across the whole study, whilst sprint times dropped by an average of one-tenth of a second. In addition, all players reported better mental and physical well-being during training and games.[11]

Here are some important factors which sleep will positively affect:

Reaction times – The smallest fraction of time will make a big difference in sport. Lack of sleep has been known to reduce this alertness and decrease reaction times. Even moderate sleep deprivation has been shown to have the same effect on reaction times as alcohol intoxication. Imagine the accuracy of scoring a penalty after a couple of beers.

Learning and memory – Sleep affects our ability to learn new tasks. Quality sleep allows our muscle memory to be ingrained, which facilitates the performance of movements without conscious control. Our focus and attention are reduced when we're sleep deprived. This makes it more difficult for us to receive new information or to tap into old information.

Motivation – In order to hit those high levels of performance, athletes must be motivated to take on whatever the day's training may be. Lack of sleep causes irritability and a loss of focus towards goals.

---

[11] Cheri D. Mah, MS, Kenneth E. Mah, MD, MS, Eric J. Kezirian, MD, MPH, William C. Dement, MD, PhD, The Effects of Sleep Extension on the Athletic Performance of Collegiate Basketball Players, *Sleep*, Volume 34, Issue 7, 1 July 2011, Pages 943–950

Hormone balance – Human Growth hormone (HGH) is an important part of the body's hormone system. It is essential for muscle repair, muscle building, bone growth, and promoting the oxidisation of fats. Most of the production of HGH happens during deep sleep, and therefore disruptions can interfere with the body's normal production of HGH and, resultantly, the recovery process.

Cortisol, also known as the stress hormone, is regulated during deep sleep as well. Cortisol levels directly impact the body's ability to digest glucose. Since endurance depends on the body's ability to metabolize glucose, which is a form of sugar that our body breaks down from the food we eat to provide energy to muscles, getting quality sleep is crucial for athletes. Glucose is the primary fuel for endurance activities like swimming, cycling, and running, where prolonged effort is required. Sleep plays a key role in energy restoration by helping the body regulate glucose levels and ensuring muscles have enough energy to sustain long periods of physical activity. Without enough sleep, the body may struggle to efficiently process glucose, leading to decreased performance and endurance.

Injury risk – Lack of sleep appears to be a big factor in injury risk. Athletes who sleep less than eight hours a night on average are approximately 1.7 times more likely to have had an injury compared with those sleeping more.[12]

Illness susceptibility – People who don't sleep for long enough or with enough quality are more likely to get ill after being exposed to a virus such as the common cold. Lack of sleep also affects how fast you recover if you do get sick. During sleep, your immune system releases

---

[12] Milewski MD, Skaggs DL, Bishop GA, et al. Chronic lack of sleep is associated with increased sports injuries in adolescent athletes. J Pediatr Orthop. 2014;34(2):129-133.
doi:10.1097/BPO.0000000000000151

chemicals such as infection-fighting antibodies which are needed for a strong immune system.

Now that you understand the importance of having good quality and quantity of sleep, here are some ways to help you improve your sleep. Just as you train to get better at your sport, you can train to improve your sleep.

Regular routine – Try to go to bed and get up at the same time every day, even if you're travelling or have a busier schedule than usual.

Avoid caffeine and alcohol – Cut out or reduce your alcohol and caffeine intake. Caffeine found in most energy drinks and coffee can seriously disrupt your sleep pattern. If going caffeine free is too difficult, then aim for a 'no caffeine after 2 pm' rule to give your body a chance to properly metabolise it before bedtime. Alcohol also has a big effect on the quality of your sleep and it decreases the healing potential of any injuries.

Limit late-night training – Vigorous workouts can raise levels of cortisol (the human stress hormone), which impairs sleep. So, scheduling an intense session right before bed may increase the time it takes to fall asleep. Sometimes this can't be helped, but try and avoid it where possible.

Drink only enough fluids to maintain proper hydration – You don't want a full bladder to keep you awake you during the night! Avoid drinking an hour before bed and remember, little and often is ideal.

Turn off the screens – TVs and smartphones emit blue light which suppresses the melatonin levels that make us sleepy. Put down the phone, turn off the TV, and keep your bedroom dark and quiet for a couple of hours before bed.

Take a nap - Naps can help you recover from a previous night of poor sleep or waking up early for a training session. But, try to avoid late-afternoon or evening naps so that you don't impact your night-time sleep routine. When you do nap, keep these to 30 minutes to avoid replacing sleep at night.

Practise relaxation techniques – These can be anything that relaxes you, from breathing techniques to light yoga. Re-read the 'fight or flight' breathing exercise chapter for a simple breathing technique to help relax you.

Avoid social media and the news – Avoiding social media and the news not only avoids blue light emitting screens, but stops your brain being stimulated. Generally, social media and the news – or even certain TV programs – will stimulate your brain. This is also exaggerated if they include anything that you don't agree with. Avoid all screens in the last couple of hours before bed; replace those that you do watch with programs that don't require much attention and are of a positive nature: this will help your body to relax before going into your sleep routine.

The Pillow Matters

One often overlooked factor that can significantly affect sleep quality is the choice of pillow. The right pillow not only helps in achieving a comfortable night's sleep but also plays a vital role in supporting the complex structures of the head, neck, shoulders, and spine. Overlooking the importance of a suitable pillow can lead to sleep disturbances, discomfort, and a variety of issues over time.

The primary function of a pillow is to keep your head, neck, and spine in natural alignment. A pillow that is too high or too soft can cause the neck to bend unnaturally, potentially straining muscles and spinal joints. On the other hand, a pillow that is too flat can lead to a downward tilt of the neck, placing pressure on the spine. Chronic misalignment can lead to neck and back pain, headaches, and long-term musculoskeletal issues.

Pillows come in various materials, each offering different benefits. As mentioned in a previous chapter, memory foam pillows, for example, are praised for their ability to contour to the shape of the head and neck, providing consistent support without losing shape. Latex pillows, which are firmer, tend to offer more support and are durable. Down or feather pillows, while extremely soft and comfortable, can compress easily and therefore may not provide adequate support for some sleepers.

Using the correct pillow can help minimise disruptions such as tossing and turning, waking up frequently, and the discomfort that can come from pressure points. The comfort of lying down on a pillow that feels *right* can create a sense of relaxation and security, which helps you to fall asleep faster. This is part of what is often referred to as 'sleep hygiene', which includes all the rituals and environmental factors that lead up to a good night's sleep.

Investing in a good pillow might seem like a small thing, but it has profound implications on your daily life and health.

Scan this QR code and within the bonus material you will find information on the proper pillows and much more, all of which I recommend and personally use!

Nutrition

Sports nutrition is a topic of constant change and research; the research continues to improve on the nutritional advice and it can sometimes feel overwhelming. I am therefore going to simply stress the importance of the correct nutrition and won't go into any specific nutrition plans. Nutrition is a subject very specific to the needs of a particular person, sport, and goals, and therefore any plans I aim to outline simply wouldn't be one-size-fits-all.

In sports and exercise, where the body is pushed to its limits and demands peak performance, the significance of nutrition as a recovery tool cannot be overstated. Proper nutrition is not only essential for fuelling athletic endeavours but also plays a pivotal role in recovery, repairing tissues, replenishing energy stores, and preparing the body for future challenges. Understanding the impact of nutrition on the recovery process is crucial for athletes aiming to optimise their performance and overall well-being.

At the most basic level, nutrition is important as it provides a source of energy and minerals required to perform and then recover to the 'normal' level. The food we eat impacts strength, endurance, performance and recovery. A nutrition plan aims to outline the right food type, energy, and nutrients to keep the body functioning at peak levels. A nutrition plan may vary day to day and month to month, depending on the specific energy demands of that period of time. Not only is the type of food important for optimal nutrition, but the times we eat throughout the day also have an impact performance levels and recovery.

If we take in more than we expel, then at the most basic level we are going to be carrying around unnecessary fuel. Furthermore, if we do not have enough of the right fuel in our bodies then we will not be able to convert the fuel into the energy. Thus, the quality of food is equally important to get right, as your body needs certain fuel for turning into particular types of energy.

Intense exercise triggers an inflammatory response in the body, which, when left unchecked, can hinder recovery and potentially lead to injuries. So, nutrition can be a powerful tool to combat inflammation. Vitamins and minerals are essential micronutrients that play an integral role in recovery. Vitamin C, for example, is vital for collagen synthesis, aiding in the repair of connective tissues. Calcium and vitamin D contribute to bone health, critical in preventing fractures and maintaining skeletal integrity. Iron supports oxygen transport to muscles, and zinc assists in immune function – both vital aspects of recovery.

To maintain a good level of sports nutrition, it normally comes down to planning and time management. If you have not got the time to plan your nutrition, then you may be a lot more likely to reach for the wrong types of food. Even if you don't go into depth when it comes to nutrition, plan what you are going to eat… you'll be surprised at the difference it will make.

Hydration

"Hydration is the process of maintaining the right volume of water and electrolytes in your body. It's the balance between fluids in and fluids out." [13]

About 60% of your body is made up of water and it plays a vital role in every bodily function. You can lose a lot of fluid when you exercise – as much as a litre or two an hour. During exercise, the main way the body maintains optimal body temperature is by sweating. Heat is removed from the body when beads of sweat on the skin evaporate, resulting in a loss of body fluid. Sweat production, and therefore fluid loss, increases with a rise in ambient temperature and humidity, as well as with an increase in exercise intensity.

---

[13] **Mosby's Medical Dictionary** (2020). *Hydration*. Elsevier

Dehydration is the process of losing more fluid than we are putting in. It is inevitable that during exercise we will cause some form of dehydration, but it is crucial that we do not cause too much of a fluid imbalance. Studies have shown that loss of fluid equal to 2% of your body mass is sufficient to cause a significant decrease in performance – that's a 1.4 kg loss in a 70 kg athlete! As dehydration occurs, there is a gradual reduction in physical and mental performance. Moreover, there is an increase in heart rate, body temperature, increased perception of how hard the exercise feels, irritability, headaches, weakness, dizziness, cramps, chills, heartburn, vomiting, and nausea.

Dehydration of greater than 2-5% loss of body weight increases the risk of serious heat related problems such difficulty in breathing, fainting, losing consciousness, or a reduction in blood volume.

Please remember that thirst is a poor indicator of dehydration: it is a delayed response. An athlete can lose over 2% of water before becoming thirsty, therefore it is important to have a strategy and understanding that stops dehydration from happening.

An athlete's level of hydration can be influenced by a lot of different factors, starting with the level, intensity, and duration of the sport. If the sport requires helmets or padding, this will increase the amount of sweating. So, ask yourself – are there regular breaks scheduled, and do you have access to fluids? For example, in sports such as football, rugby and distance running, you must consume fluids at specific times.

Another important factor in dehydration is the environment: heat and direct sun will increase the process. And remember, children are more susceptible to dehydration than adults.

I'd like to offer a general way to keep hydrated when training or competing. This is a generalised plan, so it will need to be modified depending on all of the factors I have just mentioned: your age, sport, intensity, climate, etc.

Before Exercise

- Drink about 500mls of fluid 2 hours before exercising
  Then drink a further 125-250mls immediately before exercise
  Weigh yourself

During Exercise

- Drink small amounts regularly, aiming for 125-250mls every 10-20 minutes. You can maintain optimal performance by replacing at least 80% of sweat lost during performance.

After Exercise

- You need to consume 150% of the amount of fluid lost during exercise to allow for the fluid that is naturally lost from the body. For example, if you have lost 1L of fluid, you need to drink 1.5L.
- The easiest way to calculate your fluid loss is to weigh yourself before and after training. 1kg of weight loss resulting from exercise, is roughly equivalent to 1L of fluid loss.
- This then needs to be multiplied by 1.5 to calculate the amount of fluid to consume. This does not need to be consumed all at once immediately after exercise. Aim for 500ml immediately after training, then consume the remainder at intervals afterwards.

Ice baths/Cryotherapy

Cryotherapy, which translates to "cold therapy," involves exposing the body to varying temperatures

A form of cryotherapy is Ice Baths, also called cold water immersion, and it has been a contentious subject for many years. From a personal perspective, when I played rugby and started to play at a higher level, I was always told to have an ice bath after a match. In fact, there were often wheelie bins filled up with ice in the changing rooms! If you have ever been in an ice bath then you know that it is not a nice experience. Whenever I questioned my coach, or strength and conditioning coach, as to why we were doing it, I wasn't convinced by the answers I was getting back: "It helps get rid of lactic acid", or "it's what the England rugby team are currently doing". So, when I got the opportunity at the University of Gloucestershire, I did a dissertation on the use of ice baths and ice compression machines. My conclusion was that it has its place when used in the correct way; but, if it is not done correctly, it not only slows the recovery, but can be dangerous to the long-term health of that person.

If you're interested, this is the title of my dissertation: "**A comparison of the Game Ready System™, Cold Water Immersion and no recovery modality after a Phosphate Decrement Test on male Rugby Union Players.**"

Despite its dangers in some instances, cold water immersions have become extremely popular with the rise of Wim Hof, the Ice Man.[14] It is still being researched, though, and there are several reasons why people are doing it, so let's go through a few.

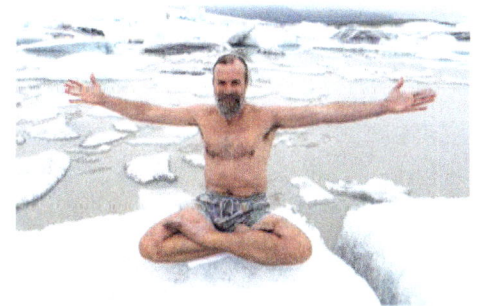

Wim Hof, the Ice Man

---

[14] https://www.wimhofmethod.com/

Cold water immersion involves immersing the body or specific body parts in cold water, typically with temperatures ranging from 10°C to 15°C for a duration of 5 to 20 minutes. The physiological responses caused by CWI contribute to its effectiveness in promoting recovery. One of the key mechanisms is vasoconstriction, which is defined by the contractions of blood vesicles for a short time; this reduces blood flow to the immersed area, thereby decreasing inflammation and tissue swelling. Additionally, the cold temperature decreases nerve conduction, leading to analgesic (numbing) effects and reducing pain perception. In further detail, CWI reduces the production of pro-inflammatory cytokines and markers of muscle damage, therefore facilitating the repair and regeneration of muscle fibers.

Numerous studies have investigated the effects of CWI on recovery from various types of exercise, including endurance, strength, and high-intensity interval training. Overall, the findings suggest that CWI can accelerate recovery by reducing muscle soreness, restoring muscle function, and enhancing performance in subsequent exercise sessions.

A meta-analysis by Hohenauer et al. (2015) demonstrated significant improvements in muscle soreness and functional recovery following CWI compared to passive rest or other recovery modalities.

Despite its potential benefits, as I mentioned earlier, CWI is not suitable for everyone. Its efficacy does vary depending on factors such as water temperature, duration of immersion, and individual reactions. Some studies have shown that the long-term effects of CWI have negative effects on muscle adaptation and performance gains. Excessive or prolonged exposure to cold water can pose risks of hypothermia, frostbite, cardiovascular stress, fertility complications, reduced protein synthesis, and reduced muscle growth, amongst others. This is particularly true in people with pre-existing health conditions or compromised thermoregulatory mechanisms. Therefore, careful assessment of the risk-benefit ratio and personalised implementation of CWI protocols are key to optimising it as a recovery strategy.

If you are thinking of using cold water immersion as a form of recovery, you must speak to a health professional to discuss the individual risk and reward for your goal in order to avoid it causing more harm than good. Gradual exposure to cold water immersion and monitoring of individual tolerance levels are essential for safety and efficacy.

Cryotherapy Chambers

The latest innovation in cold therapy is Cryotherapy Chambers. Cryotherapy chambers, sometimes referred to as cryosaunas or cold chambers, have emerged as a trendy and innovative tool for post-exercise recovery. These chambers expose individuals to extremely low temperatures for brief periods, aiming to cause similar physiological responses to cold water immersion.

Like the CWI studies, investigations into the effects of cryotherapy chambers on exercise recovery have produced conflicting results. While some research suggests significant reductions in muscle soreness, inflammation, and markers of muscle damage following cryotherapy sessions, other studies have failed to consistently demonstrate these benefits. Nonetheless, many athletes and individuals subjectively report feeling refreshed and rejuvenated after cryotherapy sessions. The variability in outcomes may come from differences in protocols, individual responses to cold exposure, and the multifactorial nature of recovery processes.

Sessions typically last only a few minutes, with temperatures ranging from -110°C to -160°C; this is obviously very cold, so there are a lot of considerations at play. Safety concerns include the risk of frostbite, cold-induced injuries, and adverse effects in vulnerable populations.

Essentially, cryotherapy chambers offer a unique approach to exercise recovery by leveraging extreme cold exposure to induce physiological responses conducive to recovery and performance enhancement. While research on their efficacy remains inconclusive, many individuals report subjective benefits from cryotherapy sessions. Understanding the mechanisms, practical considerations, and limitations of cryotherapy chamber therapy is essential for informed decision-making and safe implementation. When integrated thoughtfully into a holistic recovery regimen, cryotherapy chambers may offer athletes and fitness enthusiasts an additional tool to support their training and well-being, though the high cost of cryotherapy sessions and the lack of long-term research on their efficacy pose challenges to widespread adoption.

If you are thinking of using cryotherapy chambers as a form of recovery, you must speak to a health professional to discuss the individual risk and reward for your goal to avoid it causing more harm than good.

Compression

Compression recovery involves the use of specialised garments that control pressure on specific areas of the body, often focusing on the limbs. These compression garments come in various forms, including sleeves, socks, shorts, and full-body suits.

Compression garments apply graduated pressure to the body, causing a squeezing effect that enhances venous return and reduces the diameter of blood vessels. This compression facilitates blood flow back to the heart, thereby improving oxygen delivery to muscles and aiding in the removal of metabolic waste products accumulated during exercise. Additionally, compression garments reduce muscle oscillation and limit soft tissue movement, which may reduce muscle damage and decrease the perception of soreness. The pressure exerted by compression garments can enhance proprioception and provide a sense of stability, potentially improving neuromuscular control and functional performance.

The duration of compression garment use post-exercise varies among studies, with recommendations ranging from immediate application to prolonged wear over several hours or even days. I have found that if they fit correctly, the longer the better. In my opinion, most athletes will benefit significantly from the use of compression in recovery.

Despite the benefits, however, compression garments may not be suitable for everyone; their efficacy can be influenced by individual factors such as body composition, fitness levels, and underlying health conditions. Some people may experience discomfort or skin irritation with prolonged compression garment use.

Practical Considerations and Usage Guidelines:

Whilst the benefits of compression recovery are considerable, here are some considerations:

1. **Precise Fit and Sizing:** The correct sizing and fit of compression garments are pivotal for optimal outcomes. Ill-fitting garments may lead to discomfort or uneven pressure distribution.
2. **Graduated Compression:** Premium compression garments incorporate graduated pressure, meaning that pressure is most intense at the extremities and gradually diminishes toward the core. This graduated design is essential for promoting efficient blood circulation.
3. **Appropriate Recovery Intensity:** Compression recovery is particularly effective for mild to moderate recovery requirements. Athletes recovering from injuries should seek guidance from healthcare professionals.
4. **Trial and Personalised Response:** Each person's response to compression garments is individual. Some individuals might notice substantial benefits, whilst others may experience more modest effects. Experimenting with these garments during training can help athletes gauge response.

In this chapter we discuss the often-overlooked yet critical aspect of performance: Recovery Strategies. Recovery is the foundation upon which sustained progress is built. Without proper recovery, the body cannot heal, grow stronger, or replenish its energy reserves. This chapter explores the difference between **short-term recovery** in the immediate hours and days following an intense session, and **long-term recovery**, which must be strategically built into your training program over the course of weeks, months, or even seasons.

I have emphasised the importance of doing the simple things well – hydration, sleep, proper nutrition, and stretching – all of which are fundamental to effective recovery. Whilst advanced recovery techniques such as cryotherapy, hydrotherapy, and compression therapy can enhance the process, they are not substitutes for mastering the basics. Furthermore, recovery is about balance; overloading your body without sufficient rest will lead to breakdowns, injury, and stalled progress.

Incorporating fun elements like group recovery sessions or cross-training, as well as being mindful of proper hydration and nutrition, will help you maintain consistent and high-quality recovery. Planning your recovery with the same intention as your training is key to keeping you performing at your best.

For more information and specific recovery plans, scan the QR code; explore deeper insights and practical tools for integrating recovery into your athletic routine.

Chapter 9: Conclusion – Bringing It All Together

As we reach the final chapter of this book, I want to take a moment to reflect on everything we've explored together. Whether you identify as a Weekend Warrior, a high-level amateur, or someone who simply enjoys staying active amidst the demands of life, you now possess a comprehensive guide to improving your performance, staying healthy, and, most importantly, enjoying your journey.

Throughout the book, we've delved deep into several key areas: mindset, time management, injury prevention, recovery strategies, and training methods. We began by acknowledging the unique challenges faced by people who juggle the demands of work, family, and a passion for sport. Whilst professional athletes have the luxury of time and resources dedicated solely to their sport, you, like many others, have perhaps had to find balance. Your love for fitness and competition is driven not by external expectations, but by an internal motivation to test your limits and stay connected to the athlete within. This book is dedicated to helping you excel in your chosen pursuits, whilst ensuring that you remain injury-free and make the most of your precious time.

Mindset

At the very heart of everything we discussed is mindset. As we explored in the first few chapters, cultivating the right mindset is crucial for any athlete, but especially for Weekend Warriors. Your mental approach determines how you tackle obstacles, how you respond to setbacks, and how committed you remain to your goals even when life gets busy.

We discussed the importance of having a growth mindset, one that focuses on the process of continual improvement rather than being fixated solely on outcomes. The ability to view challenges as opportunities, rather than roadblocks, is critical for long-term success. Whether you're recovering from an injury or struggling with time management, maintaining the belief that you can improve through effort and adaptation will carry you through the tough days.

It's easy to feel disheartened when results don't come as quickly as you'd like, but remember, true progress is made over the long term. Your journey is a marathon, not a sprint. The mental strategies we discussed, like setting small, actionable goals and focusing on what you can control, will serve you well as you navigate the inevitable ups and downs of training.

Remember, it's not just about training harder; it's about training smarter. A resilient mindset keeps you grounded and focused, helping you to avoid burnout and stay the course, even when life throws challenges your way.

Time Management

One of the biggest challenges for any Weekend Warrior is time management. With a busy work schedule, family commitments, and social obligations, finding time for training can seem impossible. We explored how time management is not just about having more hours in the day... it's about prioritising and using your time wisely.

We looked at the importance of planning ahead, setting realistic goals, and creating a schedule that reflects your priorities. One of the key lessons here is that not every workout needs to be a marathon session. Consistency beats intensity in the long run. Short, focused, and intentional workouts, combined with proper recovery, can lead to significant progress over time.

In Chapter 3, we discussed practical strategies for fitting training sessions into even the busiest of days. From early morning workouts before the day begins, to squeezing in a lunchtime session, the key takeaway is that if you value your activities, you will find the time. It's all about building habits and maintaining a routine that works for you.

We also touched on the importance of balance. You don't need to train every single day to make progress. In fact, knowing when to rest is just as important as knowing when to push. Many Weekend Warriors fall into the trap of trying to cram too much training into too little time, leading to burnout and injury. Instead, by following the time management tips we covered, you can ensure that each session has a purpose, whilst still allowing time for the other important aspects of your life.

Injury Prevention

One of the core themes of this book has been the prevention and management of injuries. As someone who is passionate about sport, I'm sure you already know how frustrating it can be to be sidelined due to an injury. That's why a significant portion of this book is dedicated to helping you prevent injuries before they happen.

We explored the importance of understanding the specific demands of your sport. Whether you're a runner, cyclist, footballer, or CrossFit enthusiast, every sport places unique stress on your body. Tailoring your injury prevention strategies to these demands is crucial. By building strength, improving balance and coordination, and developing flexibility, you can reduce your risk of injury and keep doing what you love.

We also covered the importance of warm-ups and cool-downs, which many people tend to skip when they're pressed for time. These simple practices can make a world of difference in preparing your body for the stresses of training and ensuring that it recovers properly afterwards. Taking just a few extra minutes to warm up your muscles and cool down after your session can drastically reduce your risk of injury.

However, as we discussed, not all injuries are preventable. Whether due to an accident or simple wear and tear, injuries are sometimes an unavoidable part of being an athlete. When injuries do occur, the key is to respond properly. We covered the principles of rehabilitation, from the early stages of managing pain and inflammation to rebuilding strength and mobility. The importance of patience during the rehabilitation process cannot be overstated. Rushing back into training before your body is fully healed is a certain way to cause further damage and prolong your time on the sidelines.

Recovery

It's no secret that recovery is just as important as training when it comes to athletic performance. As discussed, recovery is often overlooked or neglected by people who are eager to push themselves harder and harder. However, true progress only occurs when the body has time to rest, heal, and adapt to the stresses of training.

We talked about the importance of short-term recovery in the immediate hours and days following an intense session, as well as long-term recovery, which must be built into your overall training plan. From stretching and mobility work to proper hydration, nutrition, and sleep, recovery is about more than just resting; it's about actively promoting healing and ensuring that your body is ready for the next challenge.

Proper sleep, in particular, is a game-changer. Studies have shown that athletes who get sufficient, quality sleep experience improved reaction times, better focus, and faster recovery. This is why I emphasise the importance of making sleep a priority, no matter how busy your schedule is. A good night's sleep will do more for your performance than an extra hour in the gym ever could.

And finally, we explored some of the more advanced recovery techniques that are becoming popular in the world of sports science, such as cryotherapy, hydrotherapy, and compression therapy. While these methods can certainly enhance recovery, they should always be viewed as supplements to the basics, not replacements. The key takeaway here is simple: do the simple things well, and you'll set yourself up for long-term success.

Training Methods

None of the injury prevention or recovery strategies would be complete without a focus on training methods. The training chapter provided a detailed breakdown of various approaches to improving your strength, endurance, speed, and sport-specific skills. We explored everything from strength training and cardiovascular conditioning to flexibility, mobility, and coordination.

One of the major takeaways is that your training should be diverse and well-rounded. Too many athletes fall into the trap of doing the same exercises over and over again, leading to plateaus or overuse injuries. By incorporating a variety of training methods, including cross-training and mental conditioning, you can keep your body strong, balanced, and adaptable. The more versatile your training, the better equipped you'll be to handle the challenges of your sport.

We also discussed the importance of progression. To continue improving, your training needs to evolve over time. As your body adapts to one level of stress, it's important to introduce new challenges, whether that's increasing the weight you lift, running faster, or practicing more advanced techniques. But this must always be done with an eye on proper form and safety to avoid injury and ensure steady, sustainable progress.

Your Journey as a Weekend Warrior

As I bring this book to a close, I want to speak directly to you, the reader. You're someone who has a passion for activity, sport, fitness, and the challenges that come with pushing your body and mind to their limits. You've made a commitment to yourself to continue improving, to keep competing, and to stay healthy for a long time.

But I also want to remind you that the journey of a Weekend Warrior is not just about performance metrics, personal bests, or trophies. It's about enjoying the process. Yes, you want to train hard, push yourself, and see results, but don't forget to have fun along the way. Sport and activity are about joy, camaraderie, and the love of movement. Never lose sight of that.

There will be setbacks, injuries, and challenges along the way. There will be days when you don't feel like training, when life gets in the way, and when progress seems slow. But that's okay. Remember what we discussed throughout this book: consistency, resilience, and patience are your greatest allies. Keep showing up, keep doing the work, and the results will follow.

As you move forward, take the lessons you've learned here and apply them to your unique journey. Stay committed to your goals, but also stay flexible in your approach. Be kind to your body, give it the care it needs, and above all, remember why you started this journey in the first place.

Thank you for allowing me to guide you through this process. I hope this book has provided you with the tools, insights, and confidence to continue your athletic journey with passion, purpose, and longevity. Here's to many more years of being the best version of yourself. A true Weekend Warrior.

Now, go and make it happen. "He Who Dares Wins" – Dell Boy, *Only Fools And Horses*

All the best,

Will Moore

What's next

Now that you have a load of tips and tricks that I have developed over many years of working in professional sport, it is now time to implement them. It would be unrealistic to implement all of them at once or in a short period of time. This book is meant as a guide that you can use in different situations and at different times during your sporting career. There is information in this book that you may need right now, but there is other information that you won't need for months or years. All-in-all, my aim has been to create lasting habits and strategies that you can continue to build on.

To avoid this book becoming another item on the shelf – one that hasn't been read for years – I would recommend that you re-read it on a regular basis; you don't have to read the whole book from start to finish, just skim over the chapter titles or the paragraph headings. It should take you no longer than 30 mins to skim through the whole book. This will be enough to jog your memory as to the content, and if anything does jump out that you have forgotten about, it may be relevant to you at the time of reading.

A lot of the information you need to solve a problem you will have heard before... you were just not ready to hear it at that time. For example, when your coach told you need to warm up and look after your body when you were 10 years old. At that time you had loads of energy and no aches or pains, but now, 20 years later, that advice is more relevant than ever – you're now able to hear it more clearly and take it more seriously.

The second reason we don't implement things is because we get overwhelmed – there are too many things that you would like to implement now! You try to implement everything in one go, and it is too much to stick to.

So, after a couple of weeks life gets in the way and we stop doing everything; we just go back to our normal routines. The best way to start implementing is to pick 1 or 2 things that will make the biggest difference to you, right now. They might be the easiest to do, but they are the things that will move the needle the most. When you have implemented these 1 or 2 things for a minimum of 2 weeks, then you can add 2 more strategies. A great way to keep a new habit is both via consistency and accountability, as I mentioned in previous chapters. If you implement strategies with someone else, it is easier to keep at it.

I would like to thank you for getting to the end of this book; it shows you have the passion and enthusiasm to reach your goals, whatever they may be. But don't let your journey stop here. There are a few ways in which you can continue your journey with me so that we can keep striving for whatever success looks like for you, together. Here a few ways in which you can continue your journey with me:

Free Resources: Go to https://theweekend-warrior.co.uk/warrior-resources or Scan this QR code for complimentary resources which will accompany the information you have found in this book.

Visit Moore Performance Sports Injury clinic in person or virtually: If you have a current injury or something that is holding you back from your sport, then please visit https://www.mooreperformance.uk/ for the opportunity to work with a highly skilled professional, either in person at one of our clinics, or through our virtual consultations. We'd love to see you.

To work with me personally, to request for me to speak at an event, or to talk about business development opportunities, please visit:
https://www.mooreperformance.uk/work-with-will/

References

Alison E. Field, Frances A. Tepolt, Daniel S. Yang, Mininder S. Kocher. Injury Risk Associated With Sports Specialization and Activity Volume in Youth. Orthopaedic Journal of Sports Medicine, 2019; 7 (9): 232596711987012

Brinjikji, W., Luetmer, P. H., Comstock, B., Bresnahan, B. W., Chen, L. E., Deyo, R. A., Halabi, S., Turner, J. A., Avins, A. L., James, K., Wald, J. T., Kallmes, D. F., & Jarvik, J. G. (2015). Systematic literature review of imaging features of spinal degeneration in asymptomatic populations. AJNR. American Journal of Neuroradiology, 36(4), 811–816

Cheri D. Mah, MS, Kenneth E. Mah, MD, MS, Eric J. Kezirian, MD, MPH, William C. Dement, MD, PhD, The Effects of Sleep Extension on the Athletic Performance of Collegiate Basketball Players, Sleep, Volume 34, Issue 7, 1 July 2011, Pages 943–950

International Association for the Study of Pain. (1979). Pain terms: A list with definitions and notes on usage. Pain, 6(3), 249-252

Mah, C. D., Mah, K. E., Kezirian, E. J., & Dement, W. C. (2011). The Effects of Sleep Extension on the Athletic Performance of Collegiate Basketball Players. Sleep, 34(7), 943–950

Milewski, M. D., Skaggs, D. L., Bishop, G. A., et al. (2014). Chronic lack of sleep is associated with increased sports injuries in adolescent athletes. Journal of Pediatric Orthopaedics, 34(2), 129–133. doi:10.1097/BPO.0000000000000151.

Merton, R. K. (1948). The self-fulfilling prophecy. Antioch Review, 8(2), 193–210

Mosby's Medical Dictionary. (2020). Invasive procedure. Elsevier.

Oxford English Dictionary. (2020). Habit (2nd ed.). Oxford University Press

Rosenthal, R., & Jacobson, L. (1968). Pygmalion in the Classroom: Teacher Expectation and Pupils' Intellectual Development. New York: Holt, Rinehart & Winston

Wim Hof Method. Retrieved from https://www.wimhofmethod.com/